Hypnosis House Call

A Complete Course in Mind-Body Healing

Dr. Steven Gurgevich
Foreword by Andrew Weil, MD

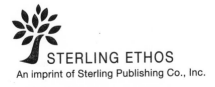

STERLING ETHOS
An imprint of Sterling Publishing Co., Inc.

New York / London
www.sterlingpublishing.com

Hypnosis House Call should not be used as a substitute for your ongoing or current medical and/or psychological therapies. If you are being treated for a mental disorder or you are in counseling, you should consult your therapist to gain professional advice about your use of self-hypnosis and this book and DVD.

The author and publisher specifically disclaim any responsibility for any liability, loss, or risk, personal or otherwise, that is incurred as a consequence, directly or indirectly, of the use and application of any of the contents of this book and DVD.

Library of Congress Cataloging-in-Publication Data
Gurgevich, Steven.
    Hypnosis house call: a complete course in mind-body healing/Steven Gurgevich.
        p. cm.
Includes bibliographical references and index.
    ISBN 978-1-4027-7747-9
    1. Hypnotism--Therapeutic use. 2. Autogenic training. 3. Mind and body. I. Title.

RC499.A8G87 2010
615.8' 5122--dc22
2010012316

10   9   8   7   6   5   4   3   2   1

Published by Sterling Publishing Co., Inc.
387 Park Avenue South, New York, NY 10016
© 2011 by Dr. Steven Gurgevich
Distributed in Canada by Sterling Publishing
^c/o Canadian Manda Group, 165 Dufferin Street
Toronto, Ontario, Canada M6K 3H6
Distributed in the United Kingdom by GMC Distribution Services
Castle Place, 166 High Street, Lewes, East Sussex, England BN7 1XU
Distributed in Australia by Capricorn Link (Australia) Pty. Ltd.
P.O. Box 704, Windsor, NSW 2756, Australia

Sterling ISBN 978-1-4027-7747-9

For information about custom editions, special sales, premium and corporate purchases, please contact Sterling Special Sales Department at 800-805-5489 or specialsales@sterlingpublishing.com.

Contents

Foreword

You are in for a treat. This book and DVD bring mind-body medicine directly to you. When Steve Gurgevich and I were growing up, doctors commonly made house calls. When you think of a house call, you don't picture the doctor examining your medical chart while you sit on a sterile, paper-covered exam table. For those who remember them, house calls centered on a warm and compassionate relationship with a trusted physician who knew and treated all the members of the family. Home visits allowed the doctor to learn a great deal about patients, their relationships, and their lifestyles. As you will read in the many case studies presented in this book, this information can help stimulate the healing process.

Steve Gurgevich is a longtime friend and colleague of mine who has specialized in mind-body medicine and clinical hypnosis for almost four decades. And, yes, he still makes house calls. *Hypnosis House Call* provides you with an opportunity to learn and experience medical hypnosis from a master.

I have been an advocate of mind-body medicine during my entire professional career, and I still practice and study its many forms. At the University of Arizona Center for Integrative Medicine, which I direct, mind-body medicine is a core subject taught to all the physicians, nurse-practitioners, medical students, and residents we train. Even though much of Western medicine still thinks of mind-body methods, including hypnosis, as merely complementary or an alternative to "real" medicine, there are now over fifty years of impressive studies that validate their central role in healing.

The new sophisticated imaging technology of positron emission tomography (PET) and functional magnetic resonance imagery (f-MRI) scans let us see the brain's activity at specific regions, correlating with specific mental states and while the patient is engaged in mind-body therapies. Studies clearly show that hypnosis is not "all in one's head" or limited to imagination and suggestion. These newer imaging technologies show the body and mind as inseparable, sharing in all experiences, both physical and mental. I hope they will help expand our understanding of health to include body, mind, and spirit. The present materialistic view that attributes physical symptoms only to physical causes severely limits our understanding of disease and our ability to treat it. Mind-body medicine concerns the nonphysical causation of changes in the body. It takes advantage of the unitary nature of mind-body to activate healing in safe, effective, and cost-effective ways, now greatly underutilized in conventional practice.

Mind-body approaches have been used throughout history. This book's appendix includes a concise history of hypnosis in medicine from ancient Greece to the modern day. Happily, the last half-century has seen an evolution of more sophisticated mind-body therapies, which are effective, inexpensive, time-efficient, and enjoyable—and without the risks associated with pharmaceutical drugs.

Hypnosis House Call is not about the research studies and is not an argument in favor of mind-body medicine. Dr. Gurgevich, or "Dr. G," as his patients call him, produced this book and DVD to share with you the benefit of learning and experiencing hypnosis for yourself. He uses a great many actual patient cases to illustrate and to enlighten the reader in much the same manner that he works with his patients. In his highly accessible house-call style, he dispels the myths and misconceptions and explains what hypnosis really is and how you can use it for healing. Readers will learn methods to induce hypnosis and discover their innate ability to experience it. Therapeutic strategies and techniques are explained in the case histories, including those where hypnosis was of limited benefit.

I know that the stories will open your eyes and mind to the powerful reality of the mind-body connection. I'm personally familiar with some of the cases, as they were patients seen in our integrative medicine clinic—teaching cases for the physicians in our fellowship training program. Others concern patients I referred to Dr. G. In fact, he has made house calls to my own home.

When my former wife, Sabine, was pregnant with our daughter, I asked Steve to do a session with her in the interest of ensuring a timely, quick, and uncomplicated birth. We were worried, because three weeks before her due date, the baby was still in a posterior presentation. Sabine's previous baby had also been posterior, which caused a long and painful labor. Steve arrived at our house in the late afternoon. During a one-hour session with comfy pillows on the living room carpet, he guided Sabine into a relaxed state of inner absorption and encouraged her to talk with the baby, asking it to turn around. He reminded mother and baby to begin enjoying their mother/daughter relationship now. And he offered posthypnotic suggestions for each of them to do what was needed for an easy labor and birth. Sabine was highly motivated, trusting, with a strong belief in the mind-body connection—an excellent hypnotic subject. After Steve guided her out of her reverie, she looked supremely relaxed. He left, and we went about making dinner. We were in the kitchen when, without warning, she bent over, clutching her belly.

"What is it?" I asked.

"I think the baby's turning," Sabine answered, amazed.

Our midwife came for dinner that night and examined Sabine. She told us that the baby had, indeed, moved to an anterior presentation, less than thirty minutes after having been asked to do so. The baby arrived right on her due date. Total labor was just over two hours—almost too brief, as we hardly had time to complete our preparations.

Witnessing "spontaneous and natural healing" achieved with hypnosis is inspiring. You will get a sense of that as well as Dr. G's compassion and dedication to empowering his patients as you invite him in for a house call.

—Andrew Weil, MD

Preface

Thank you for the opportunity to teach you how to use self-hypnosis in *Hypnosis House Call*. You will learn by reading the book and watching the DVD, then by experiencing it yourself. This book is not an academic exercise, complete with research studies intended to prove its efficacy. Instead, I put together this book and DVD to help you discover that everything you need to use hypnosis and to access your mind-body connection is already within you.

You can study the information and techniques as much as you need, in order to feel comfortable with shifting your consciousness to what is called "trance." However, if you find trance difficult to experience, it usually means you are trying too hard or are being overly analytical. Hypnosis is best learned by experiencing it. Remember what it takes to learn how to ride a bicycle? You can read about how to ride a bicycle, but it does not teach you how to actually do it. You learn to ride a bicycle when you are on the bike, it is moving, your hands are holding the handlebars, your feet are on the pedals, and you feel the balance and movement together as your body acquires the learning.

At first it seems as if there are too many things to think about all at the same time, such as steering, speed, pedals, turning. But, sooner or later, you discover that your body (or more properly, your mind-body) acquires this knowledge for you, so that today you can ride safely without having to tell your hands or feet what to do. You learned through experience—by doing it. In the same manner, you will learn how to use your inner ability to experience and apply your self-hypnosis.

Yes, it is self-hypnosis, for no one can hypnotize you any more than someone can meditate you. Others can *teach* you meditation, but they cannot *do it* to you. In this book and DVD, I use the terms *hypnosis, self-hypnosis,* and *medical* or *clinical hypnosis* interchangeably. (I also distinguish them from *stage hypnosis,* which is the nonprofessional use of hypnosis solely for entertainment purposes.) But please remember: All hypnosis is self-hypnosis, and you are in control at all times. My goal is to help you discover that you have more control of your mind-body connection than you realize. By learning and experiencing this safe, powerful mind-body method, you will be able to use hypnosis for healing, comfort, and performance enhancement.

I realize that it is easier to watch a DVD than to read a book. And I expect that you may start (or have already started) with the DVD. That's fine. I created the DVD to give you the experience of what I do in my office or clinic or when I make a hospital or house call.

I want you to know that I do not view hypnosis as an alternative to sound medical care and supervision. As a faculty member of the Arizona Center for Integrative Medicine at the University of Arizona and an advocate of integrative medicine, I encourage you to explore, evaluate, and integrate into your supervised care all healing methods that have been proven safe and effective. *Hypnosis House Call* is not a substitute for medical evaluation and treatment. Rather, it is meant to enlighten and provide you with the experience of this safe and effective mind-body healing method.

The book includes a selection of patient cases that illustrate how some of my patients—including children—have used hypnosis and the outcomes they achieved, so you can better learn ways of using it for yourself. Every person is unique, and your experience with hypnosis will be adapted to your needs and personality.

All but a few of the names and some details in the patient stories have been changed to protect their privacy. I chose cases that are good teaching examples and ones that will help you see how "natural" the process of mind-body healing can be for you. My desire is for you to be inspired by experiencing how "Everything you need is already within you."

—*Steven Gurgevich, PhD*

PART I

Hypnosis and Mind-Body Healing

*H*ypnosis House Call begins by introducing me to you. I will discuss the importance of your therapeutic rapport with this book and DVD. You will develop a foundation of information about the mind-body connection, which you will be accessing with your self-hypnosis. The more familiar you are with the mind-body connection, the greater control you will have in accessing and using the power within you. Lastly, Part I will guide you through a variety of exercises to explore your hypnotic talent and will teach you hypnotic induction methods, trance deepening techniques, and ways to alert and arouse yourself from trance.

Chapter 1

Meet the Doctor

Long before opening this book, you have had the experience of meeting a doctor or a therapist for the first time, and you undoubtedly formed important first impressions. Yet when you meet a doctor or a therapist for clinical or medical hypnosis, another vital element comes into play. That is called *therapeutic rapport,* which is the emotional bond the patient and therapist forge with each other. This rapport develops at an unconscious or subconscious level, and if the patient feels or believes that the therapist is uncertain or lacks confidence in the effectiveness of the treatment, this detracts from both their relationship and the treatment. However, if the patient feels confident in the therapist and trusts him to be competent and skilled, then that belief adds to the patient's own faith in the practitioner and certainty that together they will achieve a positive outcome.

Since I will be your doctor in this *Hypnosis House Call,* I will share information about myself so you can create an impression of me. I wish I had the opportunity to see and talk with you and learn as much as I can about you. In my clinic, of course, I have that opportunity with patients. So, in this house call, I will ask some structured, specific questions you can answer for yourself, and then I will give you some instructions on how I would use your answers to help me make hypnosis more effective for you. We call this process "tailoring," which we will cover in more detail in Chapter 12. The more personal the experience is for you, and the more personal the words, images, and ideas presented to you, the better you can relate to them and use them.

One of the first questions I would ask you is this: "What comes to mind when you hear the word *hypnosis*?" If you're like the majority of people who are unfamiliar with it, especially if you've seen the entertainment or stage version, you would answer, "It scares me." If that's true for you, you're not alone.

My very first experience with hypnosis scared me, too. One day, as a teenager in 1962, I headed home from my job as a stock boy in a bank. A few doors down from the bank was a radio station where I was able to watch a broadcast through a large window. The broadcaster was sitting at a table with a medium, a psychic, a witch, and a hypnotist. The hypnotist was a gentleman with a mustache and a goatee. At that time, it was quite spooky to me, since this style of facial hair was often reserved for scary movies and stage hypnotists. The broadcaster asked the hypnotist, "Can you hypnotize anyone?" The hypnotist turned, pointed directly at me through the window, and said, "Of course. I can even hypnotize *him*."

Who, me? No way! I flew out of the radio station. But on my way home, I stopped at the library to learn more about hypnosis. Fortunately, the librarian directed me to a two-volume set, titled *Medical Hypnosis* and written by Dr. Lewis R. Wolberg, a professor of medicine at New York Medical College. Fascinated, I checked out the books and learned about the differences between the conscious and the subconscious mind and how to mentally use words, phrases, and images to influence the mind-body connection.

When I was young, the vaccine for polio, a serious disease, was available only in the form of three injections. I was so terrified of needles that I got sick to my stomach before every shot. After my parents made me get the shots, I was even more phobic. Yet after reading Dr. Wolberg's books when I was fifteen, I was able to overcome my needle phobia by using self-hypnosis. In addition, from that time forward, I have used self-hypnosis instead of anesthesia at the dentist (see Chapter 10 for details), and also to give myself more confidence in taking tests, in overcoming shyness, in mastering other performance skills, and in enhancing healing and comfort.

I remained curious about hypnosis, and continued to read many books about it. Later, I graduated from Purdue University and then moved to the University of Arizona in Tucson, where I first received two master's degrees, and then began working toward my doctoral degree in the behavioral sciences, which included the study of clinical hypnosis. A life-changing personal experience in 1970 only encouraged me to continue these studies: I developed panic attacks, a terrifying anxiety disorder with physical symptoms that leads people to believe they are dying. These attacks are often induced by stress or a combination of stress and lifestyle factors, such as excess caffeine or lack of sleep. A cardiologist I saw about this problem assured me that I was not having a heart attack or dying. "It's only stress," he told me. It sure didn't feel like "only stress" to me! In all my studies, no one had ever mentioned or even hinted at the idea that our mind could influence our body so dramatically. With this kind of personal stake in the issue, I began learning about stress, how it affects the body, and how the mind-body connection works.

Forty years ago, this field of study, then called psychosomatic medicine, was beginning to shed light on the inseparable nature of mind and body. However, other fields of medicine still held that mind and body were separate and distinct from each other, due to the influence of René Descartes, the seventeenth-century philosopher best known for his statement, "I think, therefore I am." His belief in the separation of mind and body governed the way we thought about ourselves for four centuries. However, we now know that mind and body function in tandem. In fact, one does not exist without the other. Everything that happens within the mind has a parallel within the body, and what we experience in our body affects what we experience in our mind. Mind and body are inseparable. We use terms like *subconscious, mind-body, the mind-body connection,* or *the mind of the body,* to refer to the unity that mind and body share. I use these terms interchangeably. With self-hypnosis, I taught my mind-body to deeply relax, which, in turn, unlearned the anxiety and panic attacks. That is, I used self-hypnosis to replace anxiety with its opposite, relaxation. Little did I realize then how valuable these experiences would be in helping others with hypnosis.

In graduate school, I began studying clinical hypnosis, and after I had my doctorate, I was eligible to take professional training through the American Society of Clinical Hypnosis and the Society for Clinical and Experimental Hypnosis. These two organizations were formed by physicians in the late 1940s and 1950s to train physicians, dentists, and psychologists in the use and application of clinical hypnosis.

Since then, I have worked in a variety of hospital and clinical settings. I am clinical assistant professor of medicine at the Arizona Center for Integrative Medicine at the University of Arizona College of Medicine, and I also maintain a private practice in Tucson. Using clinical hypnosis, I have treated well over fifteen thousand patients, in sessions that number over forty thousand. I have delivered more than 200 public presentations about hypnosis and more than 120 professional presentations to my colleagues. As an active faculty member of the American Society of Clinical Hypnosis, I have now trained five-thousand-plus physicians, psychologists, and other professionals. You can see that I do not take clinical hypnosis lightly. I have devoted decades of study to developing my skills and mastering hypnosis so I can share it with as many people as I can, both patients as well as my colleagues in medicine and psychology. The book you are holding in your hands is my opportunity and privilege to teach you the powerful mind-body technique of self-hypnosis.

Chapter 2

The Beautiful Mystery of Hypnosis

Hypnosis has a wide range of applications. In my practice, I use it primarily for medical and psychological conditions and for performance enhancement. The more you know about hypnosis, the less "scary" it will be and the more comfortable you will feel practicing it. So let's now explore the beautiful mystery of hypnosis.

I do not believe anyone has a precise definition of hypnosis, but I favor the definition provided by the American Society of Clinical Hypnosis:

> **Hypnosis is a state of inner absorption, concentration, and focused attention. It's like using a magnifying glass to focus the rays of the sun and make them more powerful. Similarly, when our minds are concentrated and focused, we are able to use our minds more powerfully. Because hypnosis allows people to use more of their potential learning, self-hypnosis is the ultimate act of self-control.**

While the American Society of Clinical Hypnosis definition refers to hypnosis as a "state" of inner absorption, some other definitions refer to it as a "process" or as a "procedure" that involves a therapist and a subject. I do not think anyone has an absolute definition of hypnosis and prefer to think of it as a combination of a procedure, a process, and a state of inner absorption, with the emphasis on *inner absorption*. That is, hypnosis is a type of relaxed or passive concentration that enables us to become so absorbed and focused on our own ideas that we can exclude or minimize the energy we give to the other things going on around us. I particularly like the analogy of using our mind as a magnifying glass to focus and concentrate our ideas and thoughts so that our subconscious mind receives them clearly and accepts them.

You probably do not realize it, but you put yourself into hypnotic trances every day. You often become so inwardly absorbed and focused on your thoughts that you can ignore many of the things going on around you, even as you know they are happening. One common example is becoming so caught up in a good book or a powerful movie that you react as if it were real. But I think the best example of this kind of everyday trance is a daydream.

Think about the times when you were in a classroom as the teacher was lecturing at one end of the room and you were staring out a window. Your eyes were open and you were seeing, yet you weren't looking at what you were seeing. Your ears were also open and recording the changes in air pressure we call sound waves, so you were hearing but you weren't listening to what you were hearing. This daydreamlike state is what a hypnotic trance feels like.

But with clinical hypnosis, the difference is that you are putting yourself in a trance state deliberately, often with the help of a doctor or therapist. You have a purpose and a reason for inducing this relaxed form of focused concentration and inner absorption. It will be my role in this house call to help you experience ways to bring about the hypnotic trance for *yourself*—for all hypnosis is self-hypnosis. I cannot hypnotize anyone—and I do not believe anyone else can, either. I think that is part of the illusion promoted by stage hypnotists or by people who do not fully understand the process.

The hypnotic state we call trance is nearly identical to a daydream, and it is something you produce and experience for yourself. My role is to teach and guide you to create the state of inner absorption we call trance so you can access your mind-body connection.

Now let's look at myths and misconceptions about hypnosis.

Myths and Misconceptions

Since stage hypnotists are primarily entertainers, they often promote myths and misconceptions about hypnosis in much the same way that a magician or an illusionist wants to make it appear that magic is taking place onstage. So I would like to dispel some of the myths and misconceptions about hypnosis.

The greatest myth about hypnosis is that it is "done to someone." This is false. In over three decades of practicing clinical hypnosis, I have never "hypnotized" anyone. I cannot hypnotize you any more than I can meditate you. But I can teach you how to experience hypnotic trance, and more importantly, how to use the experience for a therapeutic or a desired outcome.

Another myth is that a person experiencing hypnosis is under the control of someone else. This is completely false. People experiencing hypnosis are *always* in control. *They* know where they are and what they are doing. *They* are in control of the experience. Here, again, therapeutic rapport is important, for the more you trust the therapist or doctor, the more likely you will be to benefit from and gain valuable insights from the experience.

Another misconception about hypnosis is that only weak-minded or gullible people can experience hypnotic trance. This also is false. My observation has been that the greater the intellect, the greater the ability with hypnosis. Sometimes people with a mental disability cannot follow the instructions or maintain enough concentration to be able to experience hypnosis, but by and large, everyone has an ability to use hypnosis to a greater or lesser extent.

The medical and psychological fields using hypnosis have developed a number of what we call "tests of hypnotizability." With them, we are able to determine how easily someone can experience hypnosis and, on that basis, we would rate the person's ability as being low or high on the scale of hypnotizability. I think perhaps a better term would be *hypnotic susceptibility* or *hypnotic talent*. It was once believed that if someone had very low talent or ability with hypnosis, he would never be able to learn it, nor do it well. However, research has shown that even people who test low on these hypnotizability scales can actually become highly hypnotizable, given a little extra time and practice.

Another misconception is that someone might not be able to come out of hypnosis. This, too, is false, for we come out of hypnosis the way we go into it, and that is by our decision and our choice. There are actually two ways we can come out of a hypnotic trance: One is by falling asleep, for sleep is not hypnosis; the other is simply choosing to come to an alert, waking state on our own.

Another myth about hypnosis is that someone could be embarrassed or would unwillingly reveal secrets. Again, this is false. At all times, the hypnotic subject is in control and would not do anything she would not ordinarily do to maintain personal integrity and well-being. If you are familiar with stage hypnosis, you might be wondering about people clucking like chickens, singing like Elvis, or doing silly, embarrassing things while in a hypnotic state. Here you have to look at the context of a stage hypnosis show. Stage hypnotists are often very skilled in the techniques and methods of influence and persuasion regarding hypnosis, and they carefully select people from the audience who are already demonstrating hypnotic phenomena, such as intense interest or being frozen with fascination about what is going on. Stage hypnotists then usually invite a group of people to the stage, and anyone accepting the invitation has already agreed to become part of the act. So, if it were a show about tap dancing or singing, anyone accepting the invitation to come on the stage would already be inclined to participate. When stage hypnotists have a group of people on the stage, they will systematically find out who has the most talent and is the most willing to participate, and then they will often work more with these volunteers. When questioned after the stage performance, people will remember what they did and also often acknowledge that they were participating based more on peer pressure to join in rather than actually being under hypnosis. (In all fairness, I will say that there are some stage hypnotists who demonstrate the value of hypnosis rather than ridicule or embarrass the volunteers.)

Keep in mind that clinical hypnosis is quite different from stage hypnosis. The goal of clinical hypnosis is not to provide entertainment and amusement to an audience. Instead, our purpose with this house call, and in the workshops I give across the country, is to use hypnosis to achieve a therapeutic outcome. We want to help our patients create their desired outcomes for health, well-being, and performance consistent with their own goals and intentions. By using this book and DVD, you will be able to do this for yourself by learning to access your own mind-body connection.

The Mind-Body Connection

In making this house call, it is important for me to tell you that your mind has two parts, which work together to make hypnosis effective for you. One part is your *conscious* mind, or what we call the "thinking" mind. Your conscious mind is that part you have trained to add and subtract and to understand the difference between a verb and a noun. It is the part of you that does your active thinking, but it is actually just a tiny part of your entire mind. The other part of the mind is called the *subconscious* mind, and this is by far the larger part of your mind, even though you do not realize it. Some people refer to it as the *unconscious,* but that reminds me of the ads for an "un-cola." *Un* tells us what something is not, rather than what it is. My preference is the term *subconscious* mind because it means that it is *sub,* or below, your conscious level of awareness.

Your subconscious mind is the mind of your body. This is an important distinction in this house call, for I will be using the terms *subconscious, mind-body,* and *mind of your body* interchangeably. Think about it: Your subconscious mind has the ability to manage your body's community of more than seventy trillion cells, and each of those cells has the capacity to maintain all the functions of life—absorption, digestion, elimination, protection, and regeneration. Your subconscious mind is able to do all this without your ever having to think about it. You do not have to think each time your body inhales or exhales. You do not have to think to manage the four chambers of your heart or your immune system or any of the other vital organs within your body. Your subconscious mind manages all these functions for you.

Your brain has the ability to create patterns to perform these and other activities automatically, and by practice and rehearsal—along with conscious desire and thoughts—you can actually create new patterns of neurons and new ways of behaving. We refer to this as *brain plasticity* or *neuroplasticity.* Until recently, it had been believed that the brain was unchangeable, but new research in neuroplasticity shows that the brain changes in accordance with our thoughts, ideas, and activities. With your hypnosis, you will actually be creating new patterns and configurations of neurons that will allow your mind and body, your conscious and subconscious minds, to share information more effectively.

In this house call, you will learn techniques about how to go into trance as the first part of learning hypnosis, but the most powerfully beneficial part of our work together will be in how you use this experience. So, for right now, remember that your mind has two parts: your conscious, thinking mind, which is reading these words and will be watching and listening to me on the DVD, and also your subconscious mind, or the mind of your body, which has the capacity to respond to what you read and hear, and most importantly, to what you allow yourself to believe.

The Language of the Subconscious

To have a better grasp of how hypnosis works, it is helpful to know that the conscious and subconscious minds do not understand language in the same way. The conscious mind can understand both literal language and more abstract speech, such as metaphors. However, the subconscious mind seems to process only literal language and because of this can often turn a figure of speech, like a metaphor, into a literal outcome in the body, as you will see later. So, when I speak to your subconscious mind, I am careful to use literal language so your subconscious mind will respond properly.

Here is an example. I am working with Hannah, who is four, and I ask her to pretend and imagine that she is riding a horse. This is how children experience trance. I would like to know her name, so I ask her, "Will you tell me your name?" She will answer my question ("Yes"), but she will not say her name. Young children are very literal-minded because their subconscious is more openly active at this stage of life than their conscious mind, and the subconscious processes only literal language. By the age of eight or nine, our minds begin to operate on a more analytically conscious level, so we can better handle abstract, figurative language.

Since the subconscious processes only literal language, I am very careful in my practice about how I use the two words *try* and *not,* and explain this to my patients. Here is why.

A coffee cup, a pencil, and a table are all concrete objects—we can touch or measure them, I can show them to you—and our conscious minds recognize that they are literally there in front of us. However, I cannot show you a *try,* and although you know what I mean, there is no object called a *try.* It cannot be measured or weighed or touched. *Try* (in the sense of making an effort, not in the sense of a court trial) is more a figure of speech because it does not exist in reality, although we use it as if it does.

Try to fall asleep. If you are not asleep in ten minutes, try harder. Ten minutes later, if you are still awake, try harder. You are not trying hard enough. Instead of getting sleepy, however, the more you try, the more you know you are awake. You will go to sleep only when you let or allow yourself to become unconscious. Or sometimes you try to remember a name; you know you know it, but no matter how hard you try to remember it, you cannot. However, if you would suggest to yourself, "I'll remember it later," as you let go of the trying, the name will more readily come to mind.

The word *try* does not mean "do." Remember Yoda from *Star Wars*? He advised Luke Skywalker, "Do or do not. There is no try." You can do something easily, quickly, slowly, comfortably, correctly, and many other ways, but you cannot "try" to do something. And your subconscious, with its very literal interpretation of language, knows it.

How would you make the word *try* literal if you were a subconscious mind? You could try a case in court, put something on trial to see whether it is this or that. So, half the time it might be this, and the other half it might be that. If you try, you are always stuck in between.

Forty years ago, when I was just learning hypnosis, I was impressed by a study in which a randomly assigned group of patients with a skin condition were given a prescription and told,

"Try this for two weeks." Another group of randomly assigned patients received the same prescription but with the instruction, "This will do it in two weeks, so use this for two weeks." The result was that the group who *tried* it had 50 percent less success in relieving their skin condition than the group who *used* it or *did* it. Learn to catch yourself saying *try* and substitute some aspect of *do*.

Another confusing figure of speech is *not*. If you are using figures of speech that the subconscious interprets in a negative way, you are going to get negative results. Like most people, you use it all the time, but in reality it literally does not exist and it does not register in your subconscious mind. When you tell yourself, "I do not want a cigarette. I do not want a cigarette," your subconscious hears, "I want a cigarette. I want a cigarette." The *not* does not register, so subconsciously you are only reinforcing your desire to smoke.

In his 1920 book, *Self Mastery through Conscious Autosuggestion,* Emile Coué wrote that when you speak affirmations to yourself, remember "never the nots," because *not* is not registered in the subconscious. Think of Gary Larson, the cartoonist who drew *The Far Side.* In his cartoon titled "What Dogs Really Hear," a woman with a dog named Ginger is saying, "Oh, mama loves you, Ginger. You're the cutest little thing, Ginger. I just think the world of you, Ginger. You're so cute, Ginger." But, in the little thought bubble above the dog's head are the words, "Blah blah blah Ginger, blah blah blah blah Ginger . . . Blah, blah blah Ginger."

In much the same way, the subconscious mind filters out and ignores the *nots*. *Not* is the absence of something rather than the presence of something else, and our subconscious mind cannot grasp that concept. Remember, the subconscious mind responds only to what is literal, to things or conditions that really do exist, and not to language that does not register the way our conscious mind might intend them to. Here is another example.

Today, 72 percent of Americans are overweight, and it is common to hear overweight people say, "I want to lose weight so badly." We know what they mean: They very much want to lose weight. But what does the subconscious mind hear? It is much like placing your order in a restaurant where the subconscious is the server:

"What would you like?"

"I want to lose weight."

"How do you want that done?"

"Badly."

"Okay. That's exactly how you will get it."

And, because the subconscious responds exactly, that is exactly what will happen. The person will lose weight *badly*, or probably not much at all. So saying you want to lose weight badly is much different than saying, "I'm losing weight easily, comfortably, and rapidly." This statement is much more positive, and your subconscious automatically will join in to help.

Remember: When you want to make changes in your life and behavior, be aware of *trying* to do something and of using words or phrases that your subconscious mind will interpret negatively. For instance, rather than use the word *try,* as in "I'm trying to stop smoking," say to yourself, "I comfortably and easily breathe only fresh, clear air now." Or, if you are in pain or have a pain disorder, rather than saying, "I don't want to hurt," say, "My body is healing deeply and comfortably."

It takes practice to change your usual pattern of thinking and come up with the correct statements for change, but even if you do it poorly at first, you will improve, and then your subconscious mind will pitch in to actually do it.

Be aware, too, of figures of speech called metaphors, which are words or phrases we use to make a comparison that is not literal. For instance, to say that someone is a snake means that this person is nasty and shifty, not a real snake. In my practice, I've found many instances over the years when metaphors used frequently by patients have been literally interpreted and manifested by their mind-bodies. For instance: She's a real pain in the neck (severe stiff neck). This has me tied up in knots (unexplained muscle spasms). He gets under my skin (terrible skin rash or acne). It makes my blood boil (extremely high blood pressure). I feel like I'm going to explode (migraine headaches). Researchers have recently found a condition they labeled "broken heart syndrome," which occurs in people, mostly women, who have recently suffered a devastating shock, such as the unexpected death of a loved one. Their hearts experience a severe weakness that mimics a heart attack: Their metaphorical broken heart becomes a literal one.

So if you are experiencing unexplained physical symptoms you would like to release, pay attention to your language. You might want to modify, or stop using, metaphors that your mind-body could interpret inappropriately. During a house call with you, I would ask about the symptoms you are experiencing and have you describe them to me. You can do this for yourself, too. Write down your symptoms and describe them for yourself. Then read what you have written. See if you can find metaphorical clues in your words and begin to change them if necessary.

You want to move from what *is* to what you would like your life *to be*. Your mind-body is available to do that for you. You do not have to figure out what your mind-body has to do, only how to conceptualize what you want in a positive manner. Your mind-body will take care of the rest.

The Three Vital Ingredients

Three vital ingredients make hypnosis effective for you: *motivation, belief,* and *expectation*. Together, they catch the attention of both your conscious and subconscious minds, which will allow you to have better success with your hypnosis. *Motivation* means wanting something, be it clearing up your skin, healing a gastrointestinal problem, or shooting a lower golf score. Next, you must *believe* that it is possible to achieve this. And finally, you must have the *expectation* that change will occur.

Here are some examples of how these three vital ingredients can work together in the mind-body connection.

Tucson, Arizona, where I live, is *hot* in the summer, often brutally hot. If you were to come to Tucson to see me, but were feeling some resistance to hypnosis, I would want to show you how powerful your mind is. I would invite you to join me outside my office when it is 105 degrees to sit in the shade of a palm tree. I would ask you to close your eyes and remember a time when you were outside someplace during a bitter cold snap. Perhaps you would remember walking across a parking lot when the wind chill was well below zero. To really get your imagination involved, I would ask you to recall how the cold and wind made your eyes water and your nose run, and how frozen your face felt in the frigid air. Then I would ask you to open your eyes and look at the goose bumps on your arm—in 105-degree heat. Perhaps your teeth would also have begun to chatter, as if you were truly in that cold environment at that moment—just by imagining it.

Here is another example of the power of the mind-body. I might ask you to recall a time at home when you saw something on the floor out of the corner of your eye and instantly jumped back. Your first impression, before you had a chance to get a good look, was that the thing on the floor was a large insect or even a small snake. Yet it turned out to be a twist tie or a piece of string or a cat toy. You reacted without conscious thought because your subconscious mind was taking good care of you and warned you immediately that you could be in danger, causing your body to go into a state of alarm in just a split second. When you got a better look, your conscious mind took over to let you know there was no danger. What is important for you to know here, is that the subconscious mind does not know the difference between what is real and what is imagined.

During a hypnotic trance, you use this same ability by creating images and ideas in your mind so that your body can respond to them as *real*. Remember those three vital ingredients of motivation, belief, and expectation? Imagine that you wanted to get rid of a wart on your hand. Your *motivation* is to have clear skin in that spot, so, first of all, the all-important motivation is there. Secondly, you create the *belief* that your skin is clear by imagining that it is already happening. You can use your mind's eye to "see" under your skin and imagine the wart's blood supply being cut off; then, just as you *expect,* it can no longer grow, and eventually it simply disappears, leaving clear, healthy skin.

The late Dr. Lewis Thomas, a legendary physician and a director of Memorial Sloan-Kettering Cancer Center in New York, was also an author. He wrote a monthly column, "Notes of a Biology Watcher," in *The New England Journal of Medicine*, and he also wrote some award-winning books. One of the chapters in his book *The Medusa and the Snail* was simply called "On Warts." In this chapter, he called warts "wonderful structures" that are actually a virus called the human papilloma virus. He went on to say that research has clearly shown how nothing works more effectively and efficiently than hypnosis to remove warts permanently. In my practice, I have seen great numbers of individuals with skin conditions, including warts (Chapter 4 contains a few of these stories), and I cannot think of a single case that did not respond positively. Again, the vital ingredients were motivation, belief, and expectation.

Hypnotic Phenomena

Hypnosis can be used to produce a wide variety of effects, or what are called hypnotic phenomena. These effects are just normal human experience, and all of them can be used therapeutically.

Here is a partial list:

- **Age progression**—imagining yourself in the future, having already attained a goal.

- **Age regression**—imagining yourself in the past so that you can better deal with a painful episode that happened long ago.

- **Amnesia**—the ability to forget.

- **Catalepsy**—the ability to effortlessly make parts of the body motionless.

- **Dissociation**—the ability to detach from the environment around you, much like imagining that you are at a beach, feeling the warm sand or hearing the waves when, in fact, you might actually be in a dental chair undergoing a procedure.

- **Hypermnesia**—the ability to remember better.

- **Hypnoanalgesia**—the ability to lessen pain.

- **Hypnoanesthesia**—the ability to entirely remove pain.

- **Ideosensory response**—the ability to combine an idea (*ideo*) with sensory experiences so that the body responds. For instance, if you simply imagine that you are holding a cut lemon close enough to smell its distinctive fragrance, your mouth automatically will pucker and begin to produce saliva. (It's likely you had this reaction by simply reading that sentence.) This happens because the mind of our body—the subconscious—cannot tell the difference between what is real and what is imaginary, so our body responds the same way to both.

– **Ideomotor response**—the ability to combine an idea (*ideo*) with an involuntary physical movement (*motor response*). By holding the idea of a word, term, or feeling in your mind, you allow your subconscious mind-body to create a way to involuntarily lift or move a finger. For example, you begin by holding the idea of *yes* in your mind, and dwelling on that idea with images of it and the feeling of *yes* (the affirmative). While holding this idea in mind, you then suggest and allow your body to create a pathway from your mind to one of your hands, so that a finger becomes energized enough to rise involuntarily (by itself). You do not select the finger that will rise or which hand the finger is on that will move. The key to an ideomotor response is that it is involuntary or happens on its own. You will be the observer. Once a *yes* finger is established, you continue on to *no* and after a *no* finger is established, you continue to include *I don't know*, or *I'm not ready to know*. By creating involuntary ideomotor movements associated individually with *yes*, *no*, and *I don't know,* these can be used to communicate with your body on a subconscious or mind-body level. Do not worry if this seems confusing now, as the examples in patient stories will make this clear.

- **Negative hallucination**—not seeing something that really is there. We actually have these quite often. Recall a time when you searched for a book, for instance, and scanned the titles on the shelf several times but could not find it. Suddenly, it seemed to jump out at you, and you noticed that it had white lettering on a black background, instead of the black lettering on a white background you were searching for. That simple color change kept your mind from noticing the words for a time.

- **Positive hallucination**—imagining that you experience something that is not really there.

- **Posthypnotic suggestion**—a suggestion offered during trance to be acted upon or experienced at a later time after trance or post-hypnosis.

- **Time distortion**—perceiving the elapsed time as shorter or longer than actual time. When you are with your lover, time has wings. When you are apart, time moves on crutches.

These phenomena happen to us every day when we are not in a deliberate hypnotic trance. Think of the times you are enjoying yourself—on a vacation, for instance—and time flies by, but when you are bored or dissatisfied, time drags. These are examples of time distortion. Or at the end of the day, you notice a bruise on your leg and do not remember how it happened until you consciously recall being in the garden and lightly bumping into a concrete bench. It was not important at the time, so you forgot about it. This is a form of hypnoanesthesia or hypnoanalgesia. And here is an everyday example of posthypnotic suggestion: When I leave for work in the morning, I see that we are out of bread and know I should pick up a loaf on the way home. I do not write it down, but make a mental note instead to remember it on my way home. Sure enough, I begin my drive home and that loaf of bread pops into my head, even though I have not consciously thought about it all day.

A note about hypnosis and children: I occasionally work with children. With them, I do not use words like *hypnosis* or *trance.* Instead, I use *pretend.* Children are excellent hypnotic subjects because they do not analyze or critique what they believe is possible. Instead, they have this marvelous capacity to use their imagination and pretend. So I would invite you to get comfortable with polishing your ability to pretend, for the greater you can pretend or *pre-intend,* the more effective your hypnosis will be.

Resistance to Hypnosis

In clinical hypnosis, *resistance* simply means the obstacles to being able to experience trance. It is natural and normal, and I expect it with everyone. I would expect you to feel resistance to many of the ideas or words or phrases you have been reading in this book or hearing on the DVD. That's fine. I make no judgments regarding any resistance you might have about doing or experiencing hypnosis for one reason: As you learn hypnosis, you will come across ideas that will challenge your current beliefs about your abilities and capabilities, so some degree of resistance is normal.

If I were to tell you that you could walk on water, you would feel a large amount of resistance, which I do not think I could overcome because I do not know how to enable you to walk on water. You might also feel resistance if I were to tell you that we can get rid of your warts or heal your irritable bowel syndrome. Or that we can open the airways of the bronchi so you can breathe better or head off an asthma attack. Or that we can help you discover a greater ability to sleep or to warm your hands or to selectively suppress your immune system so that transplanted tissue or an organ might be welcomed into your body without rejection. All these things have happened with my patients over the years.

When you have not yet experienced something that challenges your beliefs, resistance is natural. But resistance can change to acceptance when you discover what is possible, either by hearing about the experiences of others or firsthand through your own. A central goal of hypnosis is to help your subconscious mind accept ideas. For example, you can get a tooth filled without anesthesia. Initially, you may have great resistance to that belief by thinking, "No, I can't." However, once you have experienced your ability to remain comfortably relaxed during dental procedures without anesthesia, the resistance diminishes as you now believe, "Yes, I can." Henry Ford perhaps said it best: "If you believe you can or you believe you can't, you're right."

Think back to that time in your life when you knew you could not read. You could see the letters in books, but they were just meaningless marks on the page. You did not have the ability to read at that time, but with practice and guidance, you became a good reader. Now, if someone were to tell you that you cannot read, you would feel even more resistance to that idea because you know you *can* read.

In the same way, your experience with this hypnosis house call will challenge some of your beliefs about what you can heal and what you can do with the power of your mind. But as you demonstrate to yourself the power of your mind, you will begin to expand the horizons of your own capabilities. Up until about sixty years ago, it was believed that no human being could run the mile (1.6km) any faster than four minutes; common wisdom had it that this feat simply could not be done. But in 1954, Roger Bannister ran the mile in under four minutes, astonishing the world and shattering the earlier and unproven belief. Within the next six months, thirty-seven other people ran a mile in four minutes or less.

This is not an isolated case. Wilma Rudolph was born with polio, and the doctors told her that she would never walk. Her mother told her that she *would*, and Wilma chose to believe her mother. At age 16, she won a bronze medal in the 1956 Olympics in Australia, and in the 1960 Olympic games in Rome, she won three gold metals.

These cases just go to show the power of belief. So, if you feel resistance during this house call, simply be open-minded and let your resistance fade away.

Hypnotic Strategies

Two major strategies are used in clinical hypnosis: *symptomatic* and *psychodynamic.*

Symptomatic means we target the symptoms with hypnotic suggestions. If you were having a headache, we might do a lot of relaxation work. We would talk about how your head feels loose and relaxed, the muscles of your neck and shoulders are becoming more flexible, and your cheeks and jaw are relaxed. Using a symptomatic approach to a headache is much like taking two aspirin—it works with the symptoms but does not address the ultimate cause. The symptomatic approach often works very well, but when it does not, we move to a psychodynamic approach.

In the *psychodynamic* approach, we look at where the problem comes from and why the body is creating it, instead of simply treating the symptoms. Metaphors often play a role here, as in "He's a pain in the neck" for a headache or "She just burns me up" for acid reflux. I have often had patients with asthma who tell me that someone is "smothering" them or something "knocked the wind" out of them.

Realizing that you are using such metaphors can be an excellent clue to discovering the real source of your physical symptoms. Then you can change the words you use and give your mind-body a better message—one that heals instead of one that creates problems in the body.

Many times, an emotional conflict manifests as a physical symptom in the body. You might want to tell off your unreasonable boss, but you know that if you do, you could be fired and then how would you support your family? So instead of speaking up, you "stuff" or "swallow" this inner conflict and your anger. As your body acts out the truth of what you're feeling emotionally, it could show up as digestive problems.

There are times when we consciously *suppress* an emotion without much conflict between our physical and emotional selves. For instance, even if you are very sad at work and feel like crying, you choose not to cry there because you prefer to keep your sadness private. But later, at home, you let yourself cry and release the emotion. However, sometimes we *repress* our emotions without realizing it. In these cases, our subconscious takes over and does it for us. As a result, we might have a headache or develop a rash or some other symptom and not realize the connection between the symptom and our repressed emotions. To be certain you understand the distinction between suppressed and repressed emotions, think of suppression as the times you tell yourself, "I don't want to think about that." Repression is when your subconscious removes the memory from your conscious awareness for you, without your knowledge.

But now that you have begun learning about the language of the subconscious mind and figures of speech such as *try, not,* and metaphors, you can start asking yourself questions that can help you feel better when you develop various symptoms. As you ask those questions, your subconscious mind will find the best way to answer you. At that point, you will start moving to a place of more control, and be better able to release emotional conflict so that it does not turn into physical symptoms of illness.

Chapter 3

Your Experience with Hypnosis

You and I will now begin your experience with hypnosis.*
Remember, you will be safe, and you will always be
in control.

First, we will explore your hypnotic talents. We can do
this with some exercises that measure hypnotic ability.
Here are five simple methods I often use with my patients.
We can do them now, during this house call. The goal is to
use your imagination and see how well your body responds
to what you are imagining.

After doing these exercises, we'll explore ways for you to
use hypnotic induction methods—the ways you can put yourself
into a hypnotic trance—then look at ways to deepen your trance
and use hypnotic suggestions to get the results you want.

Exploring Your Hypnotic Talents

Relax and acquaint yourself with your mind-body connection.
You can stop doing any one of these if you become uncomfortable.

*The information in this chapter about hypnotic induction methods, ways to deepen your
trance, and hypnotic suggestions is based on The Self-Hypnosis Home Study Course (by
Doctor Gurgevich), with permission of Sounds True, Inc.

1. THE HAND CLASP

- Clasp your hands together and interlace your fingers. Imagine that your hands are glued together. Feel how tight the glue holds them!

- Now imagine that the glue between your hands has grown even stronger, or you can imagine that your hands are in a vise that keeps them together.

- Continue to concentrate on how firmly your hands are stuck together. Perhaps you have felt how strong super glue is. Keeping the "stuckness" firmly in mind, *try* to pull your hands apart while focusing on the image or idea of your hands stuck together.

- If your hands remain stuck to one another, let yourself play with the idea and how well your body responded to your thoughts.

- Then imagine your hands free of each other and gently pull them apart.

- If your hands did not remain stuck together, even a little, play some more and see what happens. Sooner or later, your subconscious will accept the idea and image in your mind. The key is to make the image in your mind the dominant idea as you do this.

2. THE PENCIL GRIP

- Pick up a pencil and hold it between your thumb and forefinger.

- Look at your thumb and finger holding the pencil and concentrate on them.

- Imagine that your thumb and finger press more and more tightly together, that they are a vise clamping the pencil tighter and tighter.

- Concentrate on how tightly your thumb and forefinger are gripping the pencil. Keeping the "tightness" in mind, *try* to pull them apart.

- Could you mentally "feel" that balance point where it seemed as if you could not pull your thumb and forefinger apart?

3. BUCKETS AND BALLOONS

Give your mind and body an experience of responding to opposites at the same time.

- Sit upright and hold both arms out straight in front of you.

- Imagine that one forearm has a bucket hung over it.

- Imagine that your other forearm has helium-filled balloons tied to it.

- Now picture that sand is pouring into the bucket as more helium is injected into the balloon.

- Let the bucket arm get heavier and be pulled lower, and the balloon arm get lighter and rise higher.

- Continue feeling your bucket arm get heavier and your balloon arm lighter.

- Now whenever you're ready, stop this exercise and relax both of your arms.

4. THE LEMON

This is one of my favorites. It will give you an ideosensory experience, which means that an idea in your mind (*ideo*) produces a response through your senses. Move slowly through the steps only as the images arise in your imagination.

- Imagine that you have a fresh lemon in your hand. Feel its weight as you notice its beautiful yellow color, the small dimples in the skin, its firm roundness.

- Imagine that you lightly scrape the skin to release some of the fragrant oil.

- Imagine the fresh lemon scent coming from the skin.

- Now imagine putting the lemon on a cutting board and slowly slicing it in half.

- Use your imagination to see the juice running onto the cutting board.

- Picture yourself picking up one half of the lemon and bringing it to your mouth.

- Imagine licking the juicy surface of the lemon.

Could you smell the lemon juice? Taste it? Could you feel the half-lemon in your hand?

Hypnosis Induction Methods or Going into Trance

Remember, as I mentioned earlier, neither I nor anyone else can hypnotize you. You'll find that this process becomes easier and easier with practice, and ultimately, you'll simply be able to concentrate on your intention and go immediately into the trance state.

Here are seven methods of hypnotic induction, or ways to begin going into trance. You can practice with each one to discover which ones you like best or those that are easiest for you to do. I will show induction methods on the DVD. A hypnotic induction method is simply a starting point that lets you focus your concentration in a way that allows you to make a gentle journey within. As you become familiar with "going into trance," you'll discover your own way to make this happen easily for you.

1. EYE FIXATION AND CLOSURE

- Sit upright, recline, or lie down. Choose a place above the midline to let your eyes rest upon.

- Direct your attention to that point to practice "staring."

- Once you observe that you are staring (seeing but not looking), suggest to yourself that your eyelids are becoming heavier and heavier, comfortably tired, and difficult to remain open. They may flutter. That's good.

- Let your eyelids become increasingly heavy and let them begin to close by themselves as they become heavier. If they do not begin closing in five minutes, count from ten down to zero to deepen your experience, and close them at zero.

- Let yourself rest into this comfort for as long as you like, letting go of any "trying."

- Tell yourself any suggestions or picture them as already achieved, and remind yourself that you can return to this level or deeper at future sessions as well.

- When you desire, return to a fully alert, waking state, feeling refreshed and calm.

2. PROGRESSIVE BODY RELAXATION

- Lie down or recline where you can be most relaxed.

- Close your eyes, and take and release a deep breath.

- Scan your body from head to toes (or toes to head), noticing any places of stored tension or tightness.

- From your head or toes, imagine the muscles and nerves becoming limp, loose, and relaxed.

- Create your own symbolic imagery of relaxation that conveys a message of relaxation throughout your body.

- Picture a soothing, calming color that is flowing into each limb and body part as you continue.

- Silently talk to your body and your self about relaxation, comfort, and how well your body can do this with you.

- Add a deepening technique, like counting down from ten to zero. Progressive comfort is associated with each step. Let yourself rest into this comfort for as long as you like, letting go of any "trying."

- Tell yourself any suggestions or picture them as already achieved, and remind yourself that you can return to this level or deeper at future sessions as well.

- When you desire, return to a fully alert, waking state, feeling refreshed and calm.

3. GUIDED IMAGERY

- While sitting up or lying down, close your eyes.

- Picture a "special place" or a scene of comfort and safety that you would enjoy.

- Embellish the scene with what you would hear, see, smell, feel, or taste at this place.

- Continue embellishing your imagery, choosing colors, sounds, smells, feelings, and sensations that please you.

- Create some form of vertical imagery, like a staircase, escalator, or a path down a hill. Associate this image with relaxation, comfort, and going deeper and deeper into trance.

- Use your ideas and imagery to scan your body and suggest deepening comfort and muscle relaxation.

- Let yourself rest in this comfort zone for as long as you like, letting go of any "trying."

- Give yourself relaxing suggestions or picture them as already achieved, and remind yourself that you can return to this level or a deeper level of relaxation at future sessions as well.

- When you desire, return to a fully alert, waking state, feeling refreshed and calm.

4. ARM LEVITATION

Note: If you have a neck or shoulder injury or condition, do not use this method.

- Sitting upright in a chair, extend both your arms out in front of you.

- Lower your extended arms so that just the very ends of some of your fingertips touch your knees.

- Allow your fingertips to ever-so-slightly touch your knees as your arms remain suspended.

- Imagine that one of your arms is being supported from beneath by a large balloon that is being inflated to hold more and more of the weight of your arm. You can keep your eyes open or closed, whatever makes it easier to use your imagination.

- Imagine that strings are tied along that arm from your palm to above your elbow. Notice that the strings go up and are tied to the bottom of helium-filled balloons, pulling your arm higher and higher.

- Let your arm float upward, creating your own imagery of what would make it easier and easier for your arm to continue being lighter and lighter, and rising higher and higher.

- Let your arm float up until it begins bending as it gradually moves so that a finger or thumb may touch your face.

- Allow the movements to continue until you feel your hand touch your face.

- Upon touching your face, let your arms relax into your lap and enjoy going deeper and deeper into trance.

- Let yourself rest in this comfort zone for as long as you like, letting go of any "trying."

- Give yourself any suggestions or picture them as already achieved, and remind yourself that you can return to this level or deeper at future sessions as well.

- When you desire, return to a fully alert, waking state, feeling refreshed and calm.

5. REVERSE ARM LEVITATION

Note: If you have a neck or shoulder injury or condition, do not use this method.

- Sit upright and extend either arm—it doesn't matter which one—out in front of you, so that you're looking at the back of your hand at about eye level.

- Let yourself stare at the back of your hand with your fingers pointing up.

- As you stare at the back of your hand, imagine that the handle of a small pail, like one a child would use at the beach, is going over the back of your hand.

- Picture the pail handle at your wrist and the pail hanging freely from it.

- Picture a small shovel putting shovelfuls of wet sand into the pail.

- One shovelful, two shovelfuls, and pretty soon you're seeing more sand being shoveled into the pail.

- Imagine that the pail is becoming heavier and heavier.

- Your arm is feeling the weight of the pail and your arm is being pulled down by the weight of that pail.

- Keep the picture in your mind of the wet sand in the pail now becoming heavier.

- It is becoming too much of an effort to keep your arm elevated, and it is gradually being drawn lower as the pail is becoming heavier and heavier with each additional shovelful of sand.

- Sooner or later, your arm comes all the way down to your side or to your leg, at which point the pail will then rest upon the chair or the surface next to you, and you can allow that arm to relax comfortably and completely.

- Let yourself rest in this comfort zone for as long as you like, letting go of any "trying."

- Give yourself any suggestions or picture them as already achieved, and remind yourself that you can return to this level or deeper at future sessions as well.

- When you desire, return to a fully alert, waking state, feeling refreshed and calm.

6. BREATHING AND BREATH INDUCTION

- Sitting, reclining, or lying down with your eyes closed, take three deep breaths, paying attention to any tightness or tension with each inhalation, and focusing on comfort and peace with each exhalation. With each of these three deep-breath exhalations, particularly notice the feeling of "letting go."

- Notice each exhaled breath and notice the "letting go" of the breath from your body as a means of releasing tension.

- Scan your body from head to toes (or toes to head) noticing any places of stored tension or tightness.

- Now associate each inhaled breath with gathering up some of the tension or tightness, and associate each exhalation with releasing the tension or tightness. Your in-breath gathers up tension, and your out-breath releases the tension.

- Imagine or picture waves on a seashore or something that conveys the idea of gathering and releasing.

- Each breath is now a relaxing breath.

- Associate each breath now with deepening trance. With each breath, you go deeper and deeper into a comfortable trance.

- Let yourself rest in this comfort zone for as long as you like, letting go of any "trying."

- Give yourself any suggestions or picture them as already achieved, and remind yourself that you can return to this level or deeper at future sessions as well.

- When you desire, return to a fully alert, waking state, feeling refreshed and calm.

7. THUMB AND FINGER CONDITIONED RESPONSE

- Sit, recline, or lie down.

- Close your eyes and, on your writing hand, put your thumb and forefinger together so they are touching.

- Take a great, full breath of air, and hold that breath in to the count of one to five.

- With each increasing number, notice the anxiety you are naturally and purposefully creating. As you increase the anxiety by holding your breath, make it physical by squeezing your thumb and forefinger more tightly together.

- At a count of five (time this so you are really ready to exhale), release the breath and release your thumb and forefinger, letting them part and relax.

- Remember whatever mental relaxation method or other technique of "letting go" you enjoy.

- Go into trance . . . that's it . . . just "Go into trance," remembering what it feels like for you whenever you are in trance.

- Let yourself rest into this comfort for as long as you like, letting go of any "trying."

- Give yourself any suggestions or picture them as already achieved, and remind yourself that you can return to this level or deeper at future sessions as well.

- When you desire, return to a fully alert, waking state feeling refreshed and calm.

8. RAPID INDUCTION

Once you're familiar with the induction methods, you can learn rapid induction, which relies on your intention to go quickly into a hypnotic trance. Simply set your intention to "Go into trance" and create a signal or cue to which your subconscious mind will respond by taking you into trance. For instance, when I'm at my dentist's office, I don't use any anesthesia. My dentist knows this and instead politely asks if I need a few minutes to go into trance. I tell him that if he should hit a nerve or if I get bored, that will be the cue for my subconscious to take me into a deep trance with a very pleasant numbness throughout my mouth.

Here is one rapid-induction method you might use:

- Take a deep breath and hold it, while putting your thumb and forefinger together.

- Hold your breath and squeeze your thumb and forefinger together as you look up as high as you can with your eyes.

- Let your eyelids close while you keep looking up. As you close your eyelids, release the held breath and release and relax your thumb and forefinger.

- Tell yourself that you are going into trance.

DR. G'S NO-INDUCTION INDUCTION

Finally, at some point, you will be able to use my no-induction induction. As you become familiar with going into trance, you will no longer need to use a formal induction method. Simply focus your attention on your intention to go into trance as you say to yourself, "Go into trance." And you will be there.

Alerting or Coming Out of Trance

Alerting means to come out of trance and return to a fully alert, waking state. To alert yourself, all you have to do is shift your attention to your surroundings and your intention to feeling refreshed, alert, and awake.

Then, to set the stage for a refreshing experience with this trance as well as others in the future, give yourself positive statements for feeling alert, refreshed, comfortable, and pleased. Also be sure to give yourself positive messages that will reinforce the fact that you did well with your hypnosis and that it will be easy to go into trance again.

Four Levels of Trance

There are four levels of trance, all the way from light to a deep state, similar to sleepwalking. However, the depth of your trance doesn't matter much, since most people can experience hypnotic response at all levels. Whether you are in the lightest or the deepest level, you can still respond to most suggestions. The four levels of trance are:

> **1. Light or Hypnoidal:** In this lightest level of trance, you may have some fluttering of closed eyelids, and you're aware of your surroundings, but you can mentally remove yourself from those surroundings. You will most likely be in the alpha brain-wave stage.

> **2. Medium:** You will have a greater ability to tune out your surroundings and be better able to experience a greater range of hypnotic phenomena, such as pain control, time distortion, and so on. You will be in the theta brain-wave stage.

3. Deep: You will be able to totally tune out your surroundings and alter your perception of sensory information. You will be in the theta to delta brain-wave stage, with a greater degree of being absorbed in the experience.

4. Somnambulance: This is the deepest level of trance. In this stage, you will be able to walk and perform behaviors without memories of doing so afterward. This is the stage closest to sleepwalking, with brain waves in the delta level. This is very rare, and if you experience this level, I suggest that you work with a qualified therapist, as your talent for trance lets you go very deep and your ability to go this deeply into trance interferes with "learning" it as you do it.

Ways to Deepen Your Trance

Once you are comfortable with induction methods, you can learn how to enhance and deepen your trance with these six techniques:

1. Focused attention and absorption: Find a picture or image, such as a fractal or a mandala, you can concentrate on and let yourself become more and more absorbed in it. Focusing on this image outside of yourself lets you become more absorbed in your inner experience and less aware of your surroundings. This is much like becoming absorbed in a good book or movie.

2. Vertical imagery: We talk of "going deeper" into trance, so creating mental images of the process of going deeper can help with trance. You can picture yourself riding an escalator down to lower floors (or riding up when you want to come out of trance). You can use any kind of vertical imagery as long as you associate it with deepening your trance and being absorbed in the process. This includes imagining that you are going up in a hot-air balloon as you deepen your trance. And, as the balloon returns to earth, you come out of trance.

3. Fractionation: This is the process of interrupting the trance induction repeatedly and then returning to the induction. This can be useful if you're feeling resistance to trance. It involves beginning the induction, alerting yourself to a waking state for a few moments to review the experience, and then returning to the induction. I use fractionation with patients often and describe it as becoming more and more comfortable in a pool as you're learning to swim. Each time you return to the pool, you can more comfortably go deeper as you grow more familiar with the experience.

4. Sensory enhancement: Using your senses to embellish or enhance your experience with hypnosis will make it richer and more meaningful. For example, in your trance you can imagine being at the beach, which could include hearing the waves and seagulls, feeling the wet and dry sand under your feet and the warmth of the sun on your shoulders, and watching white clouds float through a clear blue sky. Adding as much sensory detail as you can will allow you to become more absorbed in the experience of "being at the beach" and so deepen your trance.

5. Reinforcement: Giving yourself a pat on the back or acknowledging what you were able to experience or achieve will help to reinforce the skill for next time.

6. Ratification: This lets you determine how valid the trance was for you. By evaluating what you achieved, you improve your confidence and ability to proceed further, just as you did when you learned to ride a bike or swim or read.

Types of Hypnotic Suggestions

Hypnotic suggestions are the spoken or silent statements, ideas, or images in mind that convey your intention or desire to your subconscious to act on. They represent the message or idea you want your subconscious to accept as real.

Here are different kinds of hypnotic suggestions.

1. Direct suggestions are clearly and directly spoken to yourself. They are obvious to both your conscious and subconscious minds. Some examples: I am calm. I am relaxed. I am at peace. My arm is heavy. My eyelids are growing heavy.

2. Indirect suggestions are designed to bypass your conscious mind and critical evaluation. They are not easily challenged by the "critical evaluator" part of the conscious mind, yet the subconscious will easily understand and accept them. Some examples: "It doesn't matter which hand goes to sleep first." "Would you like to go into deep trance more quickly or more slowly now?"

3. Posthypnotic suggestions are offered during trance so that you can respond to them later. For example, if one of my patients was anxious about undergoing an operation, I might offer this posthypnotic suggestion: "On the day of your surgery, as you walk through the hospital door, you will immediately feel calm, relaxed, and at ease. When you are lying down, you will have all the comfort necessary to remain relaxed and at ease." Here is a posthypnotic suggestion for someone anxious about taking a test: "When I enter the classroom, I leave any worry at the door. My mind is calm and focused. I am confident that all the correct answers are within me."

4. Waking-state suggestions are statements we tell ourselves in a waking state. They include positive self-talk, affirmations, and some forms of prayer.

5. Imagery and visualization refer to holding an image in your mind during trance, which is a powerful way to offer yourself hypnotic suggestions. Since images leave so little room for interpretation, they are very powerful forms of suggestion; your subconscious accepts the pictures in your imagination very clearly and literally. For example, if you are suffering from migraines or Raynaud's phenomenon (extremely cold hands) imagine that you are wearing warm mittens, washing dishes in hot water, or sitting in a hot tub, as ways to give your subconscious (mind-body) the idea to warm your hands. The subconscious accepts the image in mind as real and acts on it by dilating blood vessels in your arms and hands, which warms them. For migraine sufferers, this directs the excess blood away from the head and into the hands. Another example: If you have a skin condition, you can imagine or picture your skin as unblemished, clear, smooth, healthy, and supple. As the subconscious accepts the idea in mind, it acts on it as if it were real and brings it about.

I think that imagery and visualization (with belief) are the most effective forms of hypnotic suggestions. They leave no room for confusion with semantics and words, as images are literal interpretations of the suggestion offered.

Three Important Messages

The Law of Dominant Effect: Whatever has dominance of your thoughts and emotions (51 percent or more of your focus) is going to have the dominant effect. This is based on the axiom that a strong emotion or belief attached to a hypnotic suggestion will replace one with a weaker belief or emotion.

The Law of Reversed Effect: The harder you try to do something, the less chance you have of achieving success. Physiological effects and changes are especially affected by this law. Imagination is much stronger than willpower. Use your imagination to evoke your own personal images instead of relying on willpower and direct suggestion entirely.

The Principle of Positive Suggestion: Positive suggestions create positive attitudes, motivations, and physiological changes. Never use the *nots* or negative suggestions.

PART II

Patient Cases of Healing

You're about to read a sampling of patient cases that illustrate how hypnosis provides healing benefits. All of them come from my practice of clinical hypnosis, which now has spanned almost four decades. The variety of cases in the following chapters shows how each person's experience with hypnosis is unique, depending on his own situation and his conscious and subconscious beliefs. Your experience with hypnosis will be individual to you as well, yet you can gather a great deal of "how to" information from reading about the experiences of other people who have used hypnosis successfully.

Many of these cases were actually house calls, but some were hospital consultations that I describe as hospital house calls. And there are a few cases presented where I did not travel to the person's home or hospital, but one of my audio recordings of hypnosis traveled to them. These are referred to as audio house calls. Additionally, there are cases from my clinical practice and teaching cases seen in my mind-body clinic at the Arizona Center for Integrative Medicine at the University of Arizona.

Two common threads run through all these cases. The first is the many ways in which stress and anxiety can manifest in the body. The second is the way in which the subconscious, or the mind-body, literally expresses the (often hidden) problem and its solution. As you read these chapters, take heart. Even though your use of hypnosis may not produce a full and final solution to a specific problem, you will be pleasantly surprised by the many other results produced by your mind-body. A medical or psychological condition may persist, but you will experience less pain, better sleep, and a greater sense of confidence and control.

The subconscious is capable of magnificent healing, particularly when we combine its inherent power with our own motivation, belief, and expectations. In each of these cases, you'll see the power and magic of belief at work—which I hope and trust will build your confidence and faith in using hypnosis for yourself.

Chapter 4

Skin: Where the Emotions Surface

The skin is the largest organ of the body. In an average adult, the skin has a surface area of about twenty-two square feet (2m²) and weighs eight to ten pounds (3.6–4.5kg). It is a wonder of biological engineering. Not only does our skin act as a container to hold all our parts together, with the fluids inside, but it is the barrier against outside organisms and prevents injury to the interior organs. It excretes waste products through perspiration. It helps us maintain our body temperature within a constant range. Each square inch (6cm²) of it contains more than a thousand nerve endings, making it a sensory organ that allows us to feel pleasure and pain.

Our skin is the part of us where we literally meet the outside world. It is also a living canvas that takes its cues from the events of our lives, as we paint on our outside some of the predominant emotions hidden inside. In decades of using hypnosis to assist people, I've participated in many powerful stories of skin healing.

Warts

Warts are a common condition that can appear anywhere on the skin. They are tiny, benign tumors of the epidermis, or top layer of the skin, caused by the human papilloma virus (HPV). While warts are not dangerous, they can be annoying and embarrassing. Typical methods of treating them include acid, scraping, or freezing, but these treatments often are not very effective in the long run. Fortunately, hypnosis is very effective in removing warts permanently, as I've seen often in my own practice.

THE BEST CHRISTMAS PRESENT

In Tucson, where I live, we like to say we can endure the hot desert summers because "It's a dry heat." Even so, when the temperature reaches 112 degrees, as it did on this day, it's *hot*—dry heat or not. Janice had brought her son, ten-year-old Kenny, to see me because of the warts on his fingers. Their dermatologist had tried all the usual treatments; they worked for a time, but the warts always returned. While Janice was very skeptical that hypnosis would eliminate them, Kenny was desperate to be rid of the embarrassing brown bumps, so she made an appointment for him to see me.

Kenny told me that he didn't want to see any more doctors about the warts. The typical treatments—freezing them with liquid nitrogen, burning them with chemical solutions—were painful and, besides, they didn't do any good.

"How would it feel for your warts to be gone forever?" I asked him.

"That would be the best Christmas present in the world!" Kenny replied, a big grin spreading across his face.

Janice and I were a little surprised by his answer, since Christmas was the furthest thing from our minds on this sweltering day, but I took Kenny's answer as a reflection of his strong motivation to rid himself of the warts once and for all. I began considering how to help him accomplish this.

When children come to me for hypnosis, I never use the word *hypnosis*. Instead, I ask them to pretend, and then I help them create stories into which I weave suggestions of how their bodies might heal.

Using visual aids can help in this process, so the first thing we did was to trace an outline of Kenny's hands on a large sheet of paper—just about every child in America has done this to create a turkey drawing for Thanksgiving. Then I asked Kenny to draw his warts on each outlined hand. He made these drawings with great attention to detail, penciling in lots of tiny dots on his paper fingers.

Now it was time to begin creating the story that would become Kenny's healing tool.

The little boy snuggled into a large, comfortable armchair, and I sat in another chair across from him. I asked him to relax and, if he wanted, to close his eyes. He did.

"Now, I would like you to imagine that you are shrinking down and down until you are so tiny that if you stood on top of your head, your hair would look like a forest to you," I said.

Kenny's expression showed that he was intent on miniaturizing himself in his mind's eye. I was glad to see that his imagination had engaged with our game of pretend.

Next, I suggested that he look for the tiny hatch on the top of his head and open it. Inside there was a ladder leading to a miniature submarine. Kenny found the hatch, and climbed down into the sub. Like any good captain, he first familiarized himself with the control panel and the steering controls. Looking through the large windshield, he began guiding his submarine down through his body, all the way to his hands.

He maneuvered the tiny sub until it was underneath one of the warts on his finger.

"Can you see roots on the wart?" I asked him. "That's where the wart takes its nutrients from your body to keep itself alive."

"Yeah, I can see them," he said, his voice relaxed but excited.

"Your submarine has little mechanical arms that you can operate," I told him, "and you can use them to snip off the roots of that wart, or maybe paint them with some kind of coating, like a rubberized coating, that would stop those roots from absorbing nourishment. Can you do that?"

Kenny had a vivid imagination, and he came up with his own solution: He put a plastic bubble around the roots, blocking their access to nourishment. To make this image even stronger, I suggested that he put a seal all around the edge of the bubble to make it extra tight. He did and then said he could see the roots wiggling because they were trying to find food but could not.

I guided Kenny to travel in his submarine to each of the warts on his hands, where he used his imagination to devise ways to prevent all the roots from getting any nutrients from his body. When the root-blocking was complete, he drove his submarine back up through his body to the top of his head, where he climbed out, went up through the hatch and closed it. When his tiny self was back on top of his head, I suggested that he return to full size, which he did, feeling satisfied with his excellent work.

As the last step, I asked Kenny to erase the warts he had drawn on the outlines of his hands, and he did a very thorough job. When I asked him if he needed the paper any longer, he said no. Our session was over.

As each month passed, Janice called to remind me that Kenny's warts had not gone away. "Hypnosis just doesn't work," she declared, her skepticism of hypnotic healing now translated into firm conviction.

As summer continued, and autumn arrived and passed into winter, she called me every month without fail. Kenny's fingers were still sprinkled with little brown warts, she reported. Each time, I gave her an "indirect suggestion" to include her in Kenny's healing. "I wonder how surprised you'll be when you discover that his warts are gone," I said.

In early January, she called again. I braced myself for more disparaging remarks. Instead, Janice told me about being in church with her children on Christmas day.

"They always sit on either side of me, and I hold whichever hand is closest," she explained. "I was holding Kenny's hand when I realized that his fingers were smooth. I whispered to him, 'Kenny, your warts are gone.' He looked up at me and, very matter-of-fact, said, 'Yeah, Mom, it's Christmas.'"

When Kenny had come to see me that previous July, did he literally mean that his warts would be gone at Christmas, giving him "the best Christmas present in the world"? His comment could just as easily have been figurative, a child simply using a common image to describe a very exciting event. What is important to understand is that his subconscious took his comment literally—as the subconscious does with everything it perceives.

Kenny was a perfect subject for hypnosis. He was strongly motivated to avoid uncomfortable and useless medical treatments in the future. He had a wonderful imagination, which enabled him to use his miniature submarine to seal off the roots of his warts to deprive them of nourishment. And he believed deeply that he had done a good job of sealing off the roots and that they would die. While he did the conscious work in my office that July day, his subconscious took over after that and did the inner work of healing to provide him with a wonderful Christmas present, right on time.

SARAH'S VOCAL CORDS

Thanks to their immense ability to imagine and pretend, children produce outstanding results with hypnosis. Sarah, who was only five when I saw her, is an excellent example. She had growths similar to warts on her vocal cords, which interfered with her ability to speak. Every month her parents took her to the hospital, where the growths would be scraped off her vocal cords while she was under anesthesia. They were worried not only about this repeated treatment itself, but about how her condition might affect her development now that she had entered kindergarten. When Sarah came from her home in Kansas to visit her grandparents—a doctor and a nurse—in Tucson, they took her to see Dr. Andrew Weil at the Arizona Center for Integrative Medicine. He was touched by Sarah's case, so he referred her to me, believing that hypnosis and mind-body methods would be much less traumatic than her monthly surgical procedures.

When Sarah and her grandmother came to my office, we all sat at the round table there. I put out some of the toys I keep on hand for my little visitors, but Sarah was not interested. Instead, she huddled in her grandmother's lap, clearly suspicious of me after all her previous trips to see doctors.

I spoke directly to Sarah, rather than to her grandmother.

"Sarah, I want you to know that our job is to work together. This will be different than seeing the doctors where you live," I said. "I am not going to even ask to examine your throat."

That seemed to reassure her, and she sat up a little straighter.

"Instead, I want to help you take control and to do the healing work yourself, using your imagination. And don't worry about the words that your doctors have used before, because there is only one word that's going to be important for us. And that word is *pretend*."

Now very curious, she leaned toward me and said, "What do I pretend?"

"It's very easy. I want you to pretend to become so, so tiny that you can take a trip inside your own body." Her eyes grew large at the idea, and she began to smile. "I'll describe your trip while you pretend. You can make this trip as much fun as you would like it to be. Are you ready to begin pretending?"

She nodded.

"Sit back in your grandmother's lap and get very comfortable," I instructed. "You can close your eyes or keep them open."

At first, Sarah kept her gaze on me as I instructed her to begin shrinking until she was so tiny she could stand on the top of her head in the forest of her hair. "The hairs are big as trees," I explained. "Begin brushing aside the leaves on the ground until you find a small door you can open."

She closed her eyes, and I asked, "Did you find the door?"

Sarah nodded. I explained that she should open the door and go down a few steps, which led to an elevator. And inside the elevator, there was an assortment of tools, including large and small scissors, paintbrushes, buckets of colorful liquids, and even laser tools, like guns and wands that she had seen in cartoons. I then explained that she would see a control panel on the wall, and it had buttons that would take her to different places in her body.

"Are you ready to take the elevator down to your throat to begin your repair work?" I asked. She nodded, so I asked, "Has the elevator stopped yet?" When she nodded again, I asked her to open the elevator doors and tell me what she saw.

When Sarah did not answer, I said, "Right there in front of you, you can see your vocal cords. They look like ropes that are strung from one side of your throat to the other. When you talk, they move to make the right sounds, but they have bumps on them that make it hard for you to talk, so the bumps need to go away. The bumps might be blue or red or pink—whatever color you like—and you can choose any of your tools to begin removing them."

Sarah's eyes remained closed and she did not speak, so after a few moments, I asked, "What are you doing?"

"I'm using a laser beam," she responded.

"Good, Sarah. Be sure you get every single one. You know, you can use any of the tools you have there with you. The laser beam is a great choice. When you put the laser beam on them, do they sizzle or shrivel up or try to protect themselves? Do they smoke?"

She remained silent, intent on her task. A few moments later, I instructed, "When you're sure you have gotten all of them, every single one, take one of those buckets of colorful liquid and use one of your paintbrushes to paint your vocal cords with it. That will protect your vocal cords from the bumps ever coming back again. Use the color that you think will be the best and the strongest."

I asked Sarah to nod when she had completed all her work and then to take the elevator back up to the top of her head and climb out. Then she could come back to her full size. Several minutes passed, and then she opened her eyes and announced, "I'm back."

To wrap up our session, I asked Sarah a variety of questions, and she told me she had found her own color to use but was otherwise silent as she sat on her grandmother's lap. After that one answer, she occasionally nodded or shook her head in response to my questions. The entire visit lasted no longer than twenty minutes.

A half-hour later, her grandmother called. "Even though Sarah didn't say much in your office, she was a real chatterbox once we got in the car," she explained. "She was so excited, telling me, 'Grandma, they were screaming, they were wiggling, they were trying to hide and get away from my laser beam, but I got every one of them. I fried them all!' She told me all the details of the noises they made and the colors that changed, and then how she coated her vocal cords with a pink paint that soaked into the ropes so that they were protected."

Obviously, Sarah had used her vivid imagination to deal strongly with the bumps on her vocal cords.

A month later, after Sarah's return home, her grandmother called me once more. Sarah's parents had taken her for the next scheduled procedure to remove the growths, but once she was anesthetized, the doctor discovered that her vocal cords were perfectly clear. No growths were visible anywhere. I heard later that her parents took her back to the hospital one more time, but during this visit, the doctor looked at her throat before the anesthesia was administered. None of the growths had returned—and in the more than twelve years since that time, Sarah's vocal cords have remained free of all growths.

Just like Kenny and his warts, which disappeared on Christmas day, little Sarah used her powers of pretending and imagination to convey the message of healing to her body, which then performed the work itself. This is a strictly symptomatic approach—we addressed only the symptoms themselves, which is often sufficient. Sometimes, however, it is necessary to probe deeper than the symptoms to look for and eliminate the cause of the condition. This is called the psychodynamic approach, and we see it clearly in Nancy's story.

BENEATH A BEARD OF WARTS

Another story about warts and healing with hypnosis has two added dimensions beyond Kenny's and Sarah's stories. One is symptom substitution, in which the outward condition disappears while the underlying cause remains, resulting in another problem surfacing. The second is that using a symptomatic approach or treating only the symptoms, as with Kenny and Sarah, sometimes is not enough. Nancy, a Catholic teenager, required deeper work to reveal the original cause of her warts, which called for a psychodynamic approach.

For about two years, Nancy had suffered with warts on her face—over two hundred of them had formed a beard and brow of warts. She had seen dermatologists throughout this time, who used all the typical wart-removal techniques of freezing, burning with chemicals, or painting them with solutions designed to make them wither and die. But nothing worked, and fifteen-year-old Nancy, formerly outgoing and pretty, was now traumatized and discouraged by her condition. When her father, Mario, brought her to see me, she frequently covered parts of her face with her hands, rarely made eye contact, and barely even smiled.

Nancy cried often and was not sleeping well, due to her distress. Mario was very sad that his daughter was suffering so much physically and emotionally. A very analytical person, employed in law enforcement, he was skeptical about hypnosis. But after a psychologist in the police department told him I had used hypnosis to help his son eliminate warts fifteen years earlier, Mario was willing to explore it. So was Nancy, who was highly motivated to have the warts permanently eradicated.

I asked her to look at a spot near the ceiling on the wall across from her, and encouraged her to stare. When she appeared to be staring, I then suggested, "Would it be all right for your eyelids to begin feeling heavier?" I continued, "And as your eyelids get heavier and heavier, your eyes will close so you can use your imagination to remove all the warts."

Within a few moments, her eyelids fluttered as they closed. I said, "That's good. Now imagine that you can see inside your body. Nod your head when you are ready to proceed." She nodded.

I asked her to imagine the warts just below the skin, to see if she could see the parts that absorbed nutrients from her body. I suggested that she begin removing them in some way. Nancy's imagination created a grinding wheel, which she described as a device that painlessly ground off the roots of the warts and vacuumed up all the tiny pieces to remove them from her body. Then she visualized painting the inside of her face a lovely pink color, applying a very dense layer of paint that prevented any nutrients from reaching the warts but maintained a healthy supply of blood flowing to her skin.

I also offered Nancy a suggestion.

"Can you imagine your immune system as having levers and knobs that you can control?" I asked.

She nodded.

"Now, find the one you can use to boost your immune system to knock the warts out of operation."

Nancy liked this idea and quickly found the right imaginary knob, which she adjusted. This was the end of her first session, and Nancy smiled as she left my office, hopeful that her warts would soon be gone.

Nancy and her father came back for a second session, so she could reinforce her imagery. As they were leaving, I asked them to contact me in a few weeks to let me know how she was doing. Mario called five weeks later to say that Nancy's face was perfectly clear. They stopped in at my office soon afterwards, and Nancy was beaming, once again a lovely girl with a clear complexion.

We had treated Nancy's warts symptomatically—that is, we had used a technique that resolved the outward symptom but had not undone its underlying cause. At the time, there had seemed no reason to do so. Yet about eight months later, I was in a grocery store when a young woman came up to me and asked if I remembered her. I didn't.

"I'm Nancy," she said. "You helped me remove my warts."

Her face was still clear and healthy-looking, yet she had gained about thirty pounds (13.5kg), which is why I hadn't recognized her. I suspected that treating the symptoms of her warts hadn't gone far enough, since gaining that much weight in so short a time is often a manifestation of an emotional problem—the literal mind of the body at work. So I asked her to tell her father to bring her back to my office.

At our next session, I knew it was important to work psychodynamically with Nancy. With her permission, I was going to help her uncover the original cause of her distress, which had first manifested itself as warts and was now expressing itself as excess weight.

"Would it be okay for your subconscious mind to give you information about where the warts came from?" I asked.

She said yes, and we first established what is called ideomotor signals, so that we could interact with her mind-body. *Ideomotor* means that an idea (*ideo*) creates a physical response (*motor*). I asked Nancy to sit upright and position her hands so that they extended beyond the arms of the chair so that her fingers could hang freely.

Then I suggested that she close her eyes. "Picture the word *yes* in your mind," I said. "See it in capital letters or written on the blackboard in yellow chalk, or imagine writing *yes* into the wet sand at the beach, or perhaps you can see *yes* lit up in lights on a sign."

I continued, saying "Let yourself *feel* the word *yes* as you imagine it. This includes *yep, yeah, uh-huh,* and every way that *yes* is expressed. As you are thinking and feeling *yes,* your body can make a pathway from your mind into one of your arms, down to your hand, and into a finger. You don't have to do anything but think *yes* and your body can energize a finger so that it can lift or twitch all by itself."

I noted that the movement of a finger could be on either hand and any finger, but she was not to try to choose which hand or which finger. It is important that the finger movement be an involuntary response. As you can see, the *idea* becomes an involuntary physical or *motor* response of a finger that is associated with *yes.*

When the index finger on her right hand quivered and lifted, I said, "That's right. And you can open your eyes and see it for yourself as you still keep thinking *yes*." Nancy was amused to see her finger gently quivering up and down.

Then I asked her to again close her eyes and cancel and erase the *yes* and now think *no* in the same manner. I gave her examples of how *no* might be pictured and felt. Within a few moments the ring finger of her left hand began to quiver and lift. I asked her to open her eyes and watch. Then I asked her to close her eyes again and to cancel and erase *no* and put the idea *I don't know* in mind. I explained, "This may also include *I don't want to know* or *I'm not ready to know*."

The pinky finger on her right hand quivered and lifted involuntarily.

When we had established the ideomotor signals, I asked Nancy to close her eyes, and then I suggested, "Is there a part of you that knows where the warts came from?" Her *yes* finger lifted. "Would it be all right for that part of you to share that information with you now?" Her *yes* finger lifted again.

"Relax and clear your mind," I continued. "Tell me when the information begins to arrive."

She began to look tense, so I said, "Continue with your eyes closed. You are safe here and I am with you. As you continue, tell me what is happening, and where this is happening."

"I'm in seventh grade," Nancy said. "Father Patrick came to our class and is telling us not to commit sins against God." Tears began to flow as she described the priest warning the girls about having sex.

"Now that your mind-body has given this information," I explained, "you can bring this information with you to as much of a waking state as needed to remain comfortable so we can talk about it and remove any bad effects. You will be able to remember it now without reliving it."

Nancy opened her eyes and remained calm as she revealed the details. (At this point, she was in a very light level of trance as she reviewed the memories available to her.) She attended a Catholic school, and one day when she was eleven or twelve, Father Patrick, her parish priest, came into the class and asked the boys to leave because he wanted to have a serious talk with the girls. He proceeded to tell the young, impressionable girls that boys have sexual impulses they cannot control, so it is the girls' responsibility to make sure they did not entice boys and lead them into sin.

This message confused Nancy at her core, although she didn't realize it at the time. As a pretty girl in her "tweens," she was beginning to develop breasts and wanted to wear makeup and do other things to make herself attractive to boys. But she also came from a strongly Catholic family who trusted their priest, and he had just informed her that it was her job to ensure that boys were not attracted to her. So her subconscious took this message literally, creating a way to keep the boys away: hundreds of warts on her face. Even after she had eliminated them, she still *subconsciously believed* she had to make herself unattractive or risk leading boys into sinning with her. Thus, she gained lots of extra weight to replace the ugly warts.

I suggested to Nancy that she look back at herself on that day when Father Patrick had made his pronouncement. Then I reminded her that she was now nearly sixteen and had a clearer idea of proper behavior between boys and girls.

"You now have control of yourself," I told her. "You don't need warts or extra weight to do that. Father Patrick did a good job of frightening you, so your subconscious mind absorbed his message and took on the job for you. But now you have all the wisdom and choices you need to maintain control of the situation. Your body doesn't need to produce any more unwanted protection, since you can do that for yourself with your conscious mind."

I asked Nancy to close her eyes and return to a place of comfort and peace within her. We then reinforced the message of her healing to her subconscious, and her yes finger responded to indicate that her deepest mind now understood. With the inner healing reinforced, I then guided Nancy to a full alert waking state with the ability to comfortably remember all that she had accomplished with her subconscious.

Within six months, Nancy had easily lost the extra weight, and her face remained free of warts. Once again, she was a lovely teenage girl, enjoying life.

Nancy's story is a powerful lesson in how the mind of the body can have a very literal response to a strong, emotional message, even without conscious awareness. However, by using hypnosis, it is possible to deliberately activate the subconscious to reverse a subconscious response to a particular stimulus and restore our health.

GUILT REVEALED AND RELEASED

Warts can also appear on the genitals. While genital warts are medically considered a sexually transmitted disease caused by the human papilloma virus, they can be prompted by an emotional response to guilt over a sexual indiscretion or a reflection of the horror of being raped. With Will, age thirty-nine, it was the former.

When warts appeared on his penis, he was quite embarrassed, and his wife was disturbed. Fortunately, before he tried any of the usual medical treatments, his family physician recommended that he use hypnosis.

In Will's session, we first established his ideomotor response with finger movements. Then I began asking questions designed to help him uncover the underlying reason for the warts.

"Is there a reason for these warts?" I asked.

His *yes* finger responded.

"Would it be okay to have that information available in our session today?"

His *I don't know* finger lifted. He was hesitant. Perhaps he wasn't ready to know or didn't want to know the origin of the warts. So I reassured him that our session was confidential and that he was safe talking with me. His *yes* finger responded by rising.

Will was a teacher. He began telling me a very emotional story about a teachers' convention he had attended in the past year, during which he had had sex with another teacher. It happened only once, but the experience left him feeling guilty, and the mind of his body produced the warts as a form of punishment.

Will's admission was a breakthrough for him. Now that he understood why the warts had appeared, he could deal with eliminating them. He was afraid that his wife would be very hurt if she knew, so I left it up to him to decide whether to confess his infidelity to her. However, he wanted to make amends with his conscience.

While he was still in trance, I asked him how he could make amends to his deeper self. His subconscious produced an image, which he described to me, of doing volunteer work at the school that he had previously declined to do.

"Perhaps your subconscious could view your dedication to doing this volunteer work as a way of making amends," I suggested to him.

Will agreed, and his *yes* finger confirmed this by rising.

"In addition, I'd like you to hold in your mind the picture of your penis being free of warts, the skin clear and smooth once again," I said.

About two months later, Will called to tell me that his warts had disappeared. He added that he had received another benefit from our session. During those weeks, he had become much more sensitive and affectionate to his wife, even asking her if they could go to counseling with the sole purpose of helping him learn how to become a more loving husband.

By transforming the energy of guilt into one of love and service, Will was able to release his subconscious need for punishment for his indiscretion, as manifested in the form of genital warts.

Shingles

Shingles is caused by the same virus that causes chicken pox. In fact, only people who have previously had chicken pox ever develop shingles, also known as herpes zoster. The virus remains dormant in the nerves affected by chicken pox, but can become active later in life. An itchy rash, which begins as red spots that later blister, shingles can be excruciatingly painful because the virus inflames nerves. This occurs along nerve pathways called dermatomes, and the rash usually appears on only one side of the body, never crossing the midline. Shingles can't be cured, but steroid creams and painkillers are prescribed to help alleviate the symptoms until the inflammation eventually disappears. From a metaphorical standpoint, shingles can be a manifestation of the expression "a thorn in my side," or simply "angry blisters."

A THORNY MARITAL SITUATION

One day I ran into Jerry, a friend of mine who practices internal medicine. He told me he had shingles, but the cortisone cream his dermatologist had prescribed was not suppressing the symptoms. A week later, I saw him again, and he wanted to tell me about an insight he'd had the night before.

While he was applying the cream to the painful rash across his ribs, his wife, Karen, said, "You know, you had those little red bumps once before."

Jerry had no memory of it. "I did?"

"Yes, you did. It happened the last time my mother called and said she wanted to come spend the winter with us, and I told her she could stay as long as she liked."

At that instant, Jerry experienced one of those "aha!" moments.

"That was it! My mother-in-law was getting under my skin," he said, expressing another insightful metaphor.

He explained that he'd had a difficult relationship with his mother-in-law and how she had "always been a thorn in my side." At the same time, he loved his wife and respected her desire to have her mother visit. Telling Karen that her mother was not welcome would hurt her feelings and make his relationship with his mother-in-law even more difficult. So he suppressed his uneasiness about the visit, but the mind of his body expressed his conflict as shingles, painting his skin with the painful rash.

Now, though, he finally understood what had happened: On the day before his shingles erupted the second time, he'd heard Karen on the phone saying, "Sure, Mom. We'd love to have you visit for as long as you'd like."

Jerry did not need hypnosis to eliminate the shingles. Once he had a conscious understanding of their underlying cause, they disappeared on their own. His mind-body had put the emotional response "out of mind," but not "out of body."

He told me that he had often referred patients to a dermatologist or treated their skin conditions himself. But, given his new insight, he said he would look deeper into their cases and ask them about circumstances in their lives that might be getting under their skin or rubbing them the wrong way.

Jerry's story is an example of how a conscious insight, whether it arrives under hypnosis or not, can eliminate a troubling symptom by restoring control to the conscious mind.

BAGGAGE AND ANGRY BLISTERS

Andrew was a retired Air Force general. At seventy-five, he was still physically fit, but his dermatologist had referred him to me for a painful case of shingles. The pain was so severe that he was not sleeping well and had to take a narcotic painkiller to be able to function at all. I took a detailed history from him and found that he had no significant stresses in his life. His wife, Suzanne, enjoyed traveling, and since his retirement, he obliged her request that he travel with her. The "angry blisters" had sprung up almost overnight after their return from a trip to Egypt.

"We had a good time," he told me. "We took a cruise on the Nile, did the usual sightseeing."

I instructed Andrew on some basic techniques of clinical hypnosis and found that he was a good subject. This is often true of people who have a higher intellect and enjoy a greater sense of self-control. While he was in trance, I offered suggestions meant to help clear up his symptoms and calm his skin and affected nerves. I also gave him an audio recording so he could practice hypnosis at home. He discovered that his pain would diminish by about a third immediately after a session. Yet the shingles did not go away, and he still couldn't sleep.

So we began working with a psychodynamic approach, searching for the underlying cause of his shingles by using the ideomotor finger signals.

With his eyes closed in a light trance, I asked, "Can you think of any reason that your body would develop shingles?"

While he replied, "None that I can think of," his *yes* finger lifted.

So I asked him a series of *yes* and *no* questions that would make it comfortable for his subconscious mind to release the cause of his shingles when he came out of trance.

When he had done so, we chatted about his recent trip to Egypt with Suzanne, who was in her seventies and had arthritis. Unable to carry her own luggage, she asked that John carry it. He understood that her physical condition made it difficult for her to carry her own bags.

"But I don't understand why she has to pack so damn much," he said. "I was in the military for thirty-two years, and I learned to pack light. But I swear she took practically all the clothes she owned."

He told me about one occasion during the trip when he was toting Suzanne's luggage and found himself so out of breath that one of the younger men on the trip offered to carry some of the bags. "I'm getting angry just thinking about it again," he said.

There was the clue. I began explaining how emotional dynamics could be expressed by his body. He did not want to deny Suzanne the opportunity to travel after she had waited so patiently for him all those years he was in the military. But he was also ready to stay home—after all, he had been away for many years. He had felt weak when he realized he could no longer carry all the luggage himself, after decades of being a general who wielded a great deal of power, both physically and professionally.

Andrew's face lit up in understanding. I suggested that he might even want to discuss the situation with Suzanne.

He called me the next morning.

"Doc, it's amazing," he said. "The shingles are just about gone."

After sleeping well for the first time in weeks, he had awakened to find that the "angry blisters" had simply disappeared. He said he felt comfortable about approaching Suzanne with a plan for future travel that would work for both of them. He now felt more in control as he began planning ways that involved her packing less so he wouldn't have to carry such heavy bags. He also thought about purchasing luggage that was easier to move.

The ex-general felt confident again. Once he realized the

problem, he was able to use his skills as a strategist to develop a workable solution, and his body responded by eliminating the shingles literally overnight.

What These Cases Teach Us

These cases show us that sometimes we only need to address the physical symptoms. This is called a symptomatic approach. But sometimes we need to use a psychodynamic approach to explore the underlying psychological or emotional cause.

Even though warts are caused by the human papilloma virus (HPV), which is a physical reality, we can use nonphysical methods of imaging and suggestion to effectively remove them. In the case of Nancy, the warts were serving a protective function, and when she used her mind to remove them, her body came up with another way to serve that purpose.

The examples with shingles also demonstrate a physical condition that may erupt from nonphysical causes. Hypnosis can be very effective in uncovering a nonphysical underlying cause (when present) for physical symptoms. And, as these cases show, once you have conscious insight or awareness of what the subconscious mind-body is literally expressing, you regain control and can choose a better way to handle the emotional factors. Sometimes that is why I encourage you to look for the metaphor your symptoms are expressing and to ask metaphorical questions. With any skin conditions, including urticaria (hives), we may ask these questions: What or who is getting under your skin? Who or what is rubbing you the wrong way? What are you itching to do? What needs to come to the surface ... or what is erupting? These metaphors beg the question: What purpose might these symptoms be serving?

Again, once you have greater awareness of what your subconscious mind-body is expressing, you can choose to express it more comfortably.

Chapter 5

Respiratory System: Breathing Easy Again

The respiratory system is that magnificent pump, a biological bellows that enables us to breathe. When our airflow is reduced rapidly and involuntarily, as in an asthma attack, we fly into a panic as the body instinctively fights not to die. That panic only worsens the situation, setting in motion a growing spiral of even less airflow and more fear. Fortunately, it is often possible to use hypnosis to retrain the body to remain calm and keep the airways open.

However, it is important to remember that asthma is a serious condition that can result from many causes. Every day in the United States, eleven people die from asthma, and emergency rooms treat five thousand people for asthma or asthma-related conditions. So, if you are going to integrate hypnosis into your medical care for asthma, select a qualified practitioner to work along with the medical supervision of your physician. Remember, hypnosis is an adjunct to medical supervision. As your symptoms improve, only alter medication upon the advice of your physician.

Asthma

BIRTHDAY BOY

In his late twenties when he came to see me, Jeff told me he had developed asthma as a child. He came to my office to see if he could use hypnosis to help reduce or eliminate this dangerous condition that was controlling his life.

Jeff was an excellent hypnotic subject, highly motivated to regain his healthy breathing. During our first session, he went into trance immediately and quickly established ideomotor signaling with a *yes* finger and a *no* finger. I asked him if it would be okay to ask him how his asthma began or what purpose it had been serving for him. His *yes* finger lifted almost before I had finished the question.

His subconscious mind took him back to the day he turned five. His mother threw him a party. He remembered being excited and rambunctious, so his mother took him aside and warned him that if he did not behave, she would send him to his room and allow his friends to enjoy the party without him. When he did not settle down, she sent him to his room alone, where he could hear the fun of his birthday celebration continuing without him. He began crying loudly, and then sobbing so hard it became difficult to breathe as mucus clogged his nose and airways. Frightened, he called for his mother, who came to his room.

She panicked when she saw him struggling to breathe and rushed him to the emergency room. The physician there reassured his mother that Jeff "only had asthma" but warned her that there would be many ER visits, every time Jeff had an asthma attack. The doctor also explained that Jeff would have to begin using a variety of medications to control the asthma.

Jeff remained calm during this entire recollection, so I then asked him to move on to his second asthma attack. It happened two years later when his family was traveling out of state. One evening when they had stopped at a motel, he heard his parents begin a loud argument. As it continued, the frightened boy heard his parents yelling that they no longer loved each other and did not want to be married. Terrified of the anger and the hateful words, Jeff began to cry, and then to sob. As his airways tightened and grew less able to take in and expel air, he began to wheeze, just as he had during his first asthma attack at his birthday party. His mother and father immediately stopped arguing to rush him to the nearest emergency room. Once again, the doctor reassured the family that Jeff simply was having an asthma attack and then handed them some medication to help restore his breathing.

The pattern of Jeff's asthma was now well-established within his own body and psyche, and within his family: They all believed he had asthma. From that time on, whenever he became severely stressed, including during painful family situations, he would have an asthma attack.

At our next session, he told me that he was now doing well, practicing his hypnosis to relax and open his airways.

"Can you show me what it's like when you have an asthma attack?" I asked.

"But I don't feel one coming on," he said.

"Your body has plenty of experience in creating asthma attacks. It's been well-trained," I insisted gently. "If you let your body do it, it will remember and create an asthma attack right here. I'm here. You have your inhaler. You'll be safe."

Jeff remained quiet but seemed to be considering my request.

"Begin slowly and carefully," I said. "See if you can reproduce some of the wheezing."

As Jeff agreed to give his body permission to produce asthma, his breathing became labored and wheezy within seconds. "Yeah, this is what it's like," he whispered, sounding amazed at how easily his body complied.

As his wheezing grew louder and his face began to turn a deep red, Jeff looked frightened. Then, very calmly, I said, "That's enough."

Instantly, his breathing became normal and quiet. He looked at me and smiled. This experience made its impact on him. Now Jeff could believe in his own ability to control his asthma. For twenty years he believed he had asthma and believed he could control it only with medicine.

In the thirty years since our sessions, I've seen Jeff a few times. I always ask him if he has had any asthma attacks. His answers are always similar.

"Sometimes when I'm stressed out, I can feel my body trying to create an attack," he says. "But then I remember that I can breathe clearly and comfortably if I choose to, so I do. My body gives up trying to start the asthma, and I've never had another attack since that one we created in your office."

Just as we unknowingly create many physical conditions for ourselves, based on our emotions and thoughts, we can also consciously "uncreate" them. Put another way, anything we learn, we can unlearn with the right combination of motivation, belief, and expectation. Once Jeff learned this important fact, he was able to put it to good use in maintaining a healthy respiratory system.

SMOTHER LOVE

Tommy was seven when his mother brought him to my office. His pediatrician had recommended that the little boy learn some relaxation and mind-body exercises to deal with a pattern of distressed breathing that his mother believed was caused by asthma. Tommy was eager to learn.

In our first session, I taught Tommy some symptomatic approaches to opening his airways, meaning he would learn to simply deal with the symptoms that occurred when it became hard for him to breathe. I often use this same approach with adults, except that with children, I don't talk about hypnosis or going into trance. Instead, I ask them to pretend, which they do very well.

I asked him to pretend he was riding a wave of air into his nostrils, and then past the sinuses, down his throat, into his windpipe, through the bronchi, and into his lungs. However, with him, I did not use these terms, but instead used *nose,* a *cave* for sinuses, and *pipes, tunnels,* and *tubes* for *trachea* (windpipe) and *bronchi.* Then I asked him to follow the exhaled air all the way back up and out along the same path. All the while, I asked Tommy to pretend to see how open and clear his airways were, and I also continued to suggest that he calm his airways to keep them open. While I was talking, Tommy began creating his own imagery so he could "see" his airways becoming more open so the air could flow in and out freely.

Even though I had suggested that he "sail" or "fly" on the air, he told me he rode a tiny surfboard on the wave of air going into his body, all the way to his lungs and back out. His airways stayed open so he could surf easily and comfortably. "And then I saw that my tummy was breathing me really easy," he said.

Next, I asked Tommy to pretend again and imagine a special place where he could go whenever he wanted to, where he was always safe and could breathe comfortably and easily. I asked him to describe this place to me.

"There are flowers," he replied. "Like those flowers that my mommy says I'm allergic to. And there'd be mac and cheese and pizza and ice cream, and stuff like that, that Mommy says I'm not supposed to eat because I'm allergic to them. Only I can have them all around me and eat all I want."

"What else is in your special place, Tommy?"

When he had described all the items in this safe place where he could breathe comfortably and easily, I asked him, "What would not be in this place?"

Instantly, out came his answer: "Mommy."

Some research literature covers "smother love" as being one of the possible causes or contributors to asthma. Tommy's answer about something that would not be in his safe place gave me the opportunity to bring his mother into his healing process. In private, I explained that, with the direction of the pediatrician, she could gradually begin introducing to Tommy the items she believed caused, or could cause, an allergic reaction in him. She should begin with very small amounts—say, one flower or one bite of food at a time—and slowly increase the amounts, while keeping a journal of his progress. In this way, she would still have a feeling of safety and control, as well as a sense of responsibility for his healing.

Then in front of Tommy, I said to her, "Your son did a great job of pretending and using his mind to open his airways."

"You did?" she asked with a smile. "What did you do?"

Tommy beamed. "I rode a surfboard, Mommy! I was on this wave of air and me and my surfboard rode all the way down into my lungs and all the way back out. I made it open real big to let us through. It was fun! I was surfing!"

Then I explained that he also imagined himself in a special safe place, and how he could use this imagery to help his body "make friends" with and adapt safely to the so-called allergens. She agreed that this was a good strategy.

In this situation, it was helpful to have both Tommy and his mother involved because she had played a mostly unconscious role in creating some of his symptom-causing beliefs about his "allergies" in the first place. Now, she could play a more positive role by staying involved in his progress in keeping his airways clear and open, and in his "making friends" with a variety of foods and environmental elements. It was necessary for her to feel that she was contributing to his healing.

Tommy's story demonstrates the benefits of using symptomatic approaches for asthma. Symptomatic approaches are valid when they allow us to train our body to respond to thoughts and ideas in ways that relax and open our airways. This method allows us to break out of the circular thought pattern in which breathing becomes difficult. This leads to anxiety, which only makes breathing even harder.

COPD

Another common respiratory condition is COPD, or chronic obstructive pulmonary disorder. A leading cause of death and illness, COPD is a group of lung diseases, such as emphysema and chronic bronchitis, in which irreversible damage to the lungs blocks airflow and makes breathing increasingly difficult.

Anxiety plays a large role in COPD, as it can in asthma. When someone cannot pull in enough air, the sympathetic nervous system releases adrenaline into the body. This causes feelings of anxiety, which disrupt the person's ability to bring in enough air, releasing even more adrenaline. So, as the body creates the physiology of anxiety, it creates a vicious circle that continues to decrease airflow.

When someone with COPD comes to see me for clinical hypnosis, I don't look for psychodynamic elements that can be healed (remember that *psychodynamic* refers to finding the origin of the problem and why the body is creating it). The lung tissue has already been clearly damaged by smoking or another cause, such as repeated infection. Instead, I offer suggestions to reduce stress and anxiety. In this way, the person can breathe more easily and more efficiently use and absorb whatever air is able to enter the lungs.

51 PERCENT DID IT

Some years ago, Phyllis came to see me about her chronic bronchitis; she had used inhalers and a variety of medications to keep it under control for decades. Except for that condition, she was healthy and robust, with an intellect that allowed her to obtain her PhD in statistics. Unfortunately, her bronchitis continued to get worse and often kept her from going to her job with a major computer corporation.

Even though she was highly motivated to be healthier, Phyllis found it difficult to accept the idea that she could use her mind to affect her airways or that stress and anxiety could aggravate chronic bronchitis. In order to increase her powers of belief, I asked her to visit my biofeedback lab, where we could measure her stress and anxiety levels as she was introduced to the techniques of relaxation with hypnosis.

During the trancework with Phyllis, I helped her imagine traveling along the airways into her lungs. I described an inhaled breath moving into her nostrils, past a moist and clear sinus, down through her nasopharynx, into her trachea, and selecting one of the clear and open bronchial tubes and then going into one lung, following the branches all the way down to the alveolar sac, where inhalation is complete. I then described riding the warmer, exhaled breath back up the bronchial tube of her lung, the warm air traveling through the clear and open bronchi, then the trachea, the nasopharynx, across the sinus, and the feeling of warm, exhaled air passing through her nostrils. (Notice the different language I used with this PhD from what I used with Tommy.) Phyllis used combinations of relaxation techniques. I added imagery that enabled her to "see" her airways being healed and her body learning and remembering all these patterns of maintaining clear and open airways.

In our sessions Phyllis asked many questions about how these techniques would work; often, she overanalyzed the techniques to the point that it was difficult for her to experience any relaxation. Then, one day in the biofeedback lab, she saw on the computer screen that her body was showing signs of a relaxation response even as she was consciously thinking about a specific trigger that had in the past led to difficulty breathing: her performance evaluation by her manager. Her next performance evaluation was coming up, and she was anticipating having the same kind of response.

Yet seeing her physical relaxation recorded on the biofeedback monitor made a big impact on Phyllis and her analytical mind. She had finally discovered that she could use the power of her mind to relax and keep her airways clear, even as she imagined future scenarios. She could now imagine herself in a stressful future situation at work—meeting with her manager for her performance evaluation—and remaining comfortably at ease and feeling positive about the outcome.

Ever curious, she asked, "How is it that I can think about my evaluation and still relax at the same time?"

"It's the law of dominant effect," I said. "That means, whatever holds the majority of your belief and emotion is what your subconscious mind will accept and act on. Even with only a few minutes of imagining your airways clear and yourself relaxed and safe during the meeting with your manager, you were able to put the dominant idea of relaxation into action." *Majority* means "more than half," so 51 percent or more does it.

When I saw Phyllis in later years, she told me that her performance evaluation had gone well—as had every one since then. She had become well-versed in using self-hypnosis to remain comfortable then, and had even begun using it in many other areas of her life. She had learned to control her chronic bronchitis to the point that it rarely bothered her again.

What These Cases Teach Us

These examples of how hypnosis can alleviate respiratory conditions show that the symptomatic approaches of visualizing, imagining, or "pretending" that airways are relaxed, open, and clear create a pattern of learning that the mind-body can memorize. With practice, the patterns can be put to use very easily, almost automatically.

In some cases, it is useful to investigate whether the breathing difficulty was learned through a strong emotional conflict or traumatic experience, as was the case for Jeff. However, in most cases, the symptomatic approach of concentrating on clear and open airways is an excellent application of using the mind-body techniques of hypnosis.

Chapter 6

Gastrointestinal System: Gut Feelings

The primary function of the gastrointestinal (GI) system is to break down food so the body can absorb its nutrients. But it's more than just a conversion canal: Science has discovered that our "belly brain," the enteric nervous system, shares close links with the brain in our head. Some emotional upsets—which may be described as "That's got me tied up in knots," "He's bugging the crap out of me," or "That's so hard to swallow"—can physically manifest as GI distress.

The Built-In Barometer

Stephanie, a woman in her early forties, came to me after a referral from her gastroenterologist. Suffering from ulcerative colitis for about seven months, she was having about twenty-five bowel movements daily, with terrible cramping and bloody diarrhea. Her gastroenterologist had insisted that it was "vital" for her to begin using steroids to control the inflammation and the debilitating symptoms that seriously interfered with her life and threatened her health. Despite a desperate desire to be healed, Stephanie resisted taking steroids. These drugs are powerful immunosuppressants that do indeed control inflammation but also suppress the immune system, which would make Stephanie susceptible to other illnesses. Other side effects include increased appetite, weight gain, and Cushing's syndrome, which produces a very round "moon face" due to fat deposits in the cheeks and neck. Stephanie was slender and attractive, and she had no desire to add these side effects to her already complex physical problems.

Since she so strongly resisted using steroids, her gastroenterologist made a deal with her. She told me, "If hypnosis doesn't help me, I promised my doctor I will take the steroids." She was very motivated.

When Stephanie came to my office the first time, I took her initial history and conducted a clinical review, as I always do with new patients. She did not report any stressful situations in her life, nor could I detect any. In fact, she had a life most people would envy, complete with a loving husband and family. Her husband had a substantial income, and Stephanie was involved in many social activities that enriched her life. But I suspected that something not yet revealed was causing her serious condition.

So I began by teaching her some techniques of self-hypnosis with suggestions targeting her symptoms. We started with an orientation about the mind-body connection and how she could use hypnosis to stimulate healing of her digestive system.

She asked, "Where do we begin?"

"By closing your eyes and turning on your imagination."

She was highly motivated to avoid taking steroids and to activate healing, and she showed signs of noticeable progressive relaxation as we continued.

"Imagine that you are traveling through the alimentary canal of your digestive system."

I then vividly described the journey from her mouth, where digestion begins with chewing, saliva, and enzymes, then swallowing, and seeing her esophagus moving the food in the proper direction. We continued through the stomach and into her small intestine, with encouragement to see the intestinal lining comfortably intact with a gentle peristalsis, or wavelike motion, that moves the food along into the large intestine or colon.

I described the journey using positive images and suggestions for healing and comfortable functioning all the way through and out the end of the alimentary canal.

I recorded the session of the hypnosis with the imagery and gave her the recording with instructions for daily practice. I asked her to return for another appointment in a week. She did, but despite using the self-hypnosis techniques, Stephanie saw no change in her symptoms. So I asked her to begin keeping a symptom journal, which is a simple process of daily recording of the date, time, and the type of symptoms experienced, their intensity and duration, and the events of the day.

She kept her journal faithfully for a week and then returned for another session. What struck me was that her symptoms did not occur around the clock. Instead, they seemed to begin around 8:30 a.m. and continue until bedtime. She had no bouts of diarrhea during the night.

"Why don't you describe your typical day to me?" I asked.

"Well, when I get up, I usually feel good," Stephanie began. "I make breakfast for Peter and the kids, and once they go off to work and school, I go down to the corral and feed the horse. He likes to eat on a very regular schedule," she added with a smile.

"But for the most part, as soon as I finish his feeding, the cramps begin. They double me over, they're so bad, and I have to make a mad dash for the bathroom. Then I'm in and out of there dozens of times the rest of the day."

"What are you generally thinking about when you feed the horse?"

"I don't really know, except that I enjoy the mornings. I look forward to getting outside and doing the chores."

We agreed that it would be helpful for her to go into a hypnotic trance and see what her subconscious could reveal about this situation. A good subject, she quickly relaxed and showed her readiness to look inward.

"Can you make any connection between your ulcerative colitis and some stress or conflict in your life?" I asked.

Her face revealed a touch of fear, and she said, "I'm afraid of something, but I don't know what, or why I should be frightened."

"You're safe here in my office, Stephanie," I reassured her. "We're just exploring any reasons for your condition. Nothing can hurt you here, and there's nothing to fear."

Her eyes closed, she nodded, and her face relaxed, so I continued. "Remember that your subconscious mind can show you where your colitis began and the reason for it."

Stephanie squirmed in her chair, looking uncomfortable and frightened again. "Whatever your subconscious reveals, remember that you're safe here and now," I reminded her. "You're in my office, so it's okay to say whatever needs to be said. You can look back in time now and describe to me what you're seeing and feeling."

"I think I'm ten," she began, "and my dad and I are out horse-back riding. We rented some horses from a stable and rode out a few miles on our own. But then, something spooked my horse! It reared up and I couldn't hold on. I fell off and broke my arm. The bone was sticking out. It looked so ugly."

Her voice wavered. "It's interesting. Now I remember that I wasn't scared very much, but the look on my dad's face—he was terrified! I'd never seen him so afraid! That scared me more than anything. He scooped me up and put me on his horse with him, and then we rushed back to the stable. We were a few miles away, so it took a while."

Stephanie's subconscious mind had just revealed a possible link between those events of decades ago and her ulcerative colitis today. I asked her now to make the emotional connection between going out to feed her horse every morning and the events of that day—specifically, her father's fear for her.

As she remained in trance, I said, "That day was many years ago. You were only ten. What happened to you was frightening, especially seeing your father so afraid for you. But now you are in your forties, and you can look back at that situation with the wisdom of your years. You can understand those events and your father's fear from an adult's perspective now, with no emotional connection that would cause your body to produce ulcerative colitis. You can easily remember that day now with total comfort and ease."

I spent a few minutes reviewing with her subconscious that she was safe today, that the event that had occurred when Stephanie was ten years old was part of her past, but not part of her present life. She came out of trance and we discussed what her subconscious had showed her. She now knew what had been "out of mind" but not "out of body."

Stephanie was astonished that she had not consciously remembered the details of the day she broke her arm, although she knew she had been aware of it in the past. She then was able to offer greater details about those circumstances: She had been very distressed and unhappy about having to wear a cast to school. I reminded her that her subconscious was now making friends with her horse of today. At that point, she remarked that her symptoms had begun soon after her family had bought their horse seven months ago. Stephanie had indeed consciously made the connection between long-ago events and her current situation.

Stephanie's condition began improving that day, and within three weeks, her symptoms had disappeared completely. She was able to feed her horse and be around him without any symptoms of her previous illness. Her subconscious mind had protected her from old traumas and frightening emotions or emotional conflicts—as it does for all of us. But when she was able to bring the old trauma to light as an adult and understand it as an adult, she was able to see that her subconscious mind-body no longer had any reason to hold on to the childhood fear.

Stephanie came back to see me six years later, again referred by her gastroenterologist. Her old symptoms had returned, and knowing how well it had worked for her in the past, he suggested hypnosis for her once again. She told me in a matter-of-fact way that she was still happy with her life. She was proud of her oldest son, who had recently left home for his freshman year in college. But one of her sisters had breast cancer, and their mother had also had it.

"Do you think there might be some connection for you with your son leaving home and your mother and sister having breast cancer?" I asked. "Or perhaps you're afraid that you might also develop cancer?"

"No," she said in a straightforward voice. "No. I don't think that's true."

So we proceeded with hypnosis. While she was in trance, I asked her to let her subconscious mind review her life at that time, while reminding her that it was safe to reveal her emotions about anything. She began to cry softly as her conscious defenses came down, and she admitted being afraid that she might also develop breast cancer. Yet as her subconscious allowed this fear to surface, she also revealed another event that seemed to be much more significant to her recurrence of ulcerative colitis, which had begun during the previous Christmas holidays.

Her son had come home for Christmas break, his first visit back since moving out of state to attend college. During dinner one evening, he announced proudly that he had been elected president of his school's gay student union. This was the first time he had told his family that he was gay, yet everyone in the family accepted the news well. Stephanie's husband was not surprised in the least, having believed for many years that his son was gay. Outwardly, Stephanie was not surprised either, and was proud of her son for being elected president of the organization.

Yet subconsciously, her fear began to grow—she knew how difficult life could be for a gay man in America, and although she worried about her son's safety and happiness, she was not able to express these fears consciously. However, her body felt these underlying fears and brought back her earlier symptoms.

Once these hidden feelings surfaced, Stephanie realized that her mind-body had once again protected and shielded her by expressing the emotional stress with physical symptoms. From that day on, her symptoms have not returned. She now understands that she has a built-in barometer for emotional stress hidden from her conscious awareness. I've found this "barometer" to be common among people who are good subjects for hypnosis. Their subconscious mind often builds heavy protective walls around painful subjects that then find a physical way to express in the body.

Triggered by Plaid

A bank teller named Jenna was referred to me by her gastroenterologist because he could not find an organic basis for her nausea and vomiting problem. Like Stephanie, she showed no signs of overt stress; she enjoyed her job, and she appeared very happy with her family and her life in general. But she had developed episodes of acute nausea and vomiting. These symptoms occurred only while she was at work, which forced her to leave for the rest of the day. When it began happening on a frequent basis about two years earlier, it jeopardized not only her job but her well-being.

In our first session, I taught her some relaxation exercises embedded with specific hypnotic suggestions meant to address her nausea. I also asked her to keep a symptom journal for the next two weeks.

During that time, she came for two more appointments. At neither appointment could she identify any stress in her life that could be causing her symptoms. She was using self-hypnosis to relax well enough, but when she was at work, she was still having episodes of nausea and vomiting. When we reviewed her symptom journal, we saw that two words appeared on every day she became violently nauseated: *plaid shirt*.

"Plaid shirt?" I asked. "Does that mean anything to you?"

"No, I don't think so," Jenna answered. "I was just following your instructions to write down everything that was going on when I noticed the nausea start."

So we did some trancework to see if her subconscious would reveal the connection between the nausea and plaid shirts. Even before I finished asking the question, Jenna became hysterical. Trembling and perspiring, she was nearly screaming in fear. "The gun . . . I'm going to die!"

"Jenna, remember that you're in my office and you're completely safe here," I gently reminded her. "Remember that you are now forty-one, that your life is going well. You are safe."

Calmer now, she began to tell the story that her subconscious mind was allowing to be revealed. In vivid detail, she described a robbery at her bank two years earlier. One of the bank robbers carried a shotgun that he held to her head as he instructed everyone else in the bank to lie on the floor while one of his accomplices hurriedly stuffed money into bags. Terrified, Jenna believed she would die and never see her husband and children again. At this point in revealing her story to me, Jenna's subconscious mind offered a crucial detail: The man with the shotgun was wearing a plaid flannel shirt.

"What happened when it was all over?" I asked.

"I ran to the bathroom and threw up," she immediately replied.

Since then, every time a man wearing a plaid flannel shirt came into the bank, the sight of him triggered her suppressed terror of the robbery, and she became violently nauseated for reasons she could not explain. Her conscious mind had buried this detail of her terrifying experience until she went into trance and her subconscious understood that it could now safely reveal it. We worked to reframe that experience.

In psychology, to *reframe* something means to change the perspective through which we view it, much like changing a photograph in a frame. While we cannot alter the photo itself, we can change the frame that holds it so that we can experience it in a different way. We reframed Jenna's experience of the robbery to one she had successfully survived, so that her body no longer had to protect her with nausea and vomiting. Both her conscious and subconscious minds could now identify plaid flannel shirts with clothing she and her family enjoyed wearing, and any connections between that type of shirt and the bank robbery would be reserved specifically to thoughts of that event.

Without realizing it, Jenna had been suffering from PTSD, or post-traumatic stress disorder. With PTSD, it is common for any internal or external cues resembling aspects of the trauma—like the robber's plaid shirt—to trigger the emotions of the trauma or to make the sufferer relive the trauma all over again. So I provided Jenna with some brief counseling for her PTSD, and her symptoms quickly eased and resolved.

What's So Hard to Swallow?

Matt was referred to me by his corporate employer's medical director. The young engineer was having difficulty swallowing, and none of the examinations or tests by a gastroenterologist, a neurologist, or an ear, nose, and throat specialist had found any physical reason for his condition. We refer to this condition as *globus hystericus,* which means it is a nonphysical or psychological "lump in his throat." He was also prone to experiencing symptoms of gagging, as well as nausea and vomiting, while at work or when under stress. Nothing was organically wrong with his throat or esophagus, yet Matt would often gag while trying to swallow food or liquids. This had been going on for about two months.

During our clinical interview in his first visit, Matt told me he was engaged to his high school sweetheart, who still lived in Milwaukee; he had moved to Tucson for his job. To begin, I taught him some self-hypnosis for relaxation. He found this helpful at work and his symptoms diminished, yet he continued to have some problems with swallowing. He described the sensation to me, saying, "It feels like I have a lump in my throat."

So we did some trancework. While in trance, I asked Matt the metaphorical question, "Would it be all right to find out what is so hard for you to swallow?"

Matt began to cry and I reminded him, "I am with you and it is okay to cry and let it out, but tell me what is causing the tears. You can now remember the details consciously and speak about this to me."

"I was on the phone with Amy two months ago," he said. "I'd been missing her and told her I could hardly wait for our wedding and her move to Tucson. But she said we should see other people." His voice trailed off, and I waited for him to continue.

"Then she said flat out that our engagement was over, she was no longer engaged to me, and she would mail the ring back to me soon. I told her I would collect it from her the next time I go back home."

After some gentle questioning, he said he had never been able to fully acknowledge that he would never marry his cherished sweetheart. He told me he could not express his sorrow in words, but often had felt a lump in his throat instead. During his first session with me, just a few weeks earlier, he had spoken about his engagement very positively, not confiding at that time that Amy had broken it off.

Matt came out of trance. Even after the trancework, it was difficult for him to talk about the end of his engagement, as he could barely say anything without crying and becoming choked up. We had one more session during which he became able to talk about the situation while remaining calm. The lump in his throat disappeared, and he was able to swallow perfectly once again.

Matt's case reminded me of an old quote: "The sorrow which has no vent in tears may make other organs weep" (Henry Maudsley, prominent English psychiatrist 1835–1918).

Just Do It!

Sister Margaret, a Catholic nun, is also a hospital microbiologist. When she was a missionary in South America, she contracted a serious gastrointestinal illness that eventually required surgical intervention; this created an ileostomy. Her small intestine was attached to the abdominal wall to bypass the large intestine so that digestive waste exits through an artificial opening into a small bag. The surgery was successful, but Sr. Margaret had experienced digestive problems ever since then, and she often had to undergo an endoscopy.

This procedure requires the patient to swallow a very thin tube that has a tiny camera and other tools attached to the end of it. The camera sends video pictures during its journey to the stomach; the doctor can also use the other tools to take small tissue sections for biopsy. Patients are usually given a light sedative to reduce gagging and distress during this uncomfortable procedure.

Sr. Margaret came to me to learn hypnosis in hopes that it would relieve her digestive problems. Yet, unlike most of my patients, she had great difficulty learning how to let herself enter a pronounced state of relaxation. Later, I came to realize that, as a microbiologist, she has to be extremely analytical and to exercise extreme care in her work scrutinizing cells under a microscope. With the kind of diagnostic testing they do, microbiologists, including Sr. Margaret, have no margin for error; they must follow all procedures precisely. Should they make a mistake, it could have grave consequences for the patient whose cells they are examining.

Many microbiologists are attracted to this work in the first place because they are precise and analytical people. Hypnosis requires the ability to let go of intellectual explanations, which microbiologists find hard to do. The desire to overanalyze the process causes the learning process to take longer. This was the case with Sr. Margaret, who is indeed very intellectual and analytical.

After eight sessions, Sr. Margaret believed she had not truly experienced trance. Then she had to undergo another endoscopy, a procedure she dreaded because it caused her great discomfort. Yet she came to her next appointment with a big smile on her face.

Sr. Margaret was always pleasant during our sessions, but never had she been this happy. "What happened?" I asked.

"I just had another endoscopy," she announced, "and I decided to use my self-hypnosis."

"That's great, Sr. Margaret. From that smile, it looks like the procedure went well."

"It did! When they were going to start the IV with the sedative, I said that I would rather use self-hypnosis to relieve my discomfort and stay calm. I swallowed the endoscope, and had no trouble at all during the entire exam."

"Congratulations!"

"I was alert and attentive the whole time. I even watched it on the video monitor. Afterward, there was no need for me to go to the recovery room, and I was able to drive myself home."

Her successful experience taught Sr. Margaret that she could use hypnosis effectively without having to be in a deep trance or without having a deeply altered consciousness. She became a firm believer in self-hypnosis, and still uses it for many applications.

A Buried Psychic Wound

I made a hospital-house call to see Nina, a three-hundred-pound (136kg) woman who was hospitalized with "belly pain" from suspected recurrent pancreatitis. She was very sweet and soft-spoken, and her way of speaking was almost childlike. For twenty years she had experienced multiple hospitalizations for her recurrent pain, and despite surgery to remove her gallbladder and appendix, her intense pain recurred.

She described her pain to me, saying, "It feels like a knife stabbing me in the core of my belly."

Nina was married to a trucker who was on the road much of the time, and they lived in a rural mountain area of Arizona. They had no children. Her gastroenterologist was familiar with my work with hypnosis and suspected that her pain might be more emotional in origin than physical.

Nina was open and eager to learn self-hypnosis. In the first session she relaxed and all her pain went away.

"I'm amazed!" she said. "I can't believe that my pain is gone."

I told her I would return to the hospital to see her in the morning.

The following morning, Nina told me she had had nightmares and had spent the night crying, instead of vomiting as before.

We did another session of hypnosis and during the trance-work I asked, "Is there a part of you that knows where the pain is coming from?"

In a few moments, Nina came out of trance and was in tears. We spent time talking. I learned that her mother had died when she was very young, and she grew up with her father. He ran a roadside fruit and vegetable stand in the Midwest and would allow customers to have sex with Nina, who was about eleven or twelve at that time, for money. This revelation made clear the depth of her psychic wounds, which would not be resolved with hypnosis alone.

After many years of suffering pain, obesity, and depression, Nina was referred to inpatient psychiatric therapy, where she received intense treatment. She made a wonderful recovery and began her new life free from the burdens of her past.

What These Cases Teach Us

The digestive system and the alimentary canal (starting at the mouth, and continuing through the stomach, the intestines, to the anus) is highly sensitive and reactive to stress, anxiety, and emotions. Most of us are familiar with the feeling of having "butterflies" in our stomach before giving a performance, or just looking at something and thinking, "That makes me sick." Perhaps this greater sensitivity is due to the number of nerves and blood vessels connecting the brain and the digestive system. I am not sure of the reason, but I have observed the expression of symptoms in the digestive tract with greater frequency than those expressed in other functional systems of the body. And we see some of the highest rates of "placebo response" for digestive system drugs being tested in clinical trials, meaning that the mind exerts a great deal of influence over GI function.

The cases in this chapter illustrate how stress and anxiety may become expressed as physical symptoms without one's awareness, and how useful hypnosis is in alleviating those symptoms. In all but one case, we see that the subconscious produces symptoms that protect the person from the distressing emotions of earlier-life events. Finding the "triggers" for their symptoms involved using hypnosis to access the mind-body connection in order to ask questions and retrieve information that was "out of mind, but not out of body." And even though the physical symptoms were distressing and uncomfortable, we see that they served a protective or useful purpose in shielding the sufferer from emotional distress, whether past or present.

In the case of Sr. Margaret, I wanted to show that when hypnosis is approached from an overly analytical perspective, it is more difficult and takes longer to learn. In her case, when she chose to "just do it" and not think about it, she discovered a key feature of learning hypnosis. That is, you learn hypnosis and trance by experiencing it. I often say during the trancework, "You make it happen by letting it happen."

Chapter 7

Cardiovascular System: The Heart of the Matter

The heart was once believed to be the home of the mind; later, the brain was assigned that designation. Today, however, groundbreaking research has demonstrated that the heart contains a nervous system sophisticated enough to qualify as a "heart brain." Researchers have confirmed that the heart is much more complex than formerly believed, able to maintain two-way communications with the entire body. Unexpressed emotion can affect the heart severely; *broken heart* is an apt metaphor.

Drowning in Tears

Early in my career as a psychologist, I met with Thomas, who was hospitalized and near death from severe hypertension and congestive heart failure. Because of his heart failure, his heart could barely pump blood through his body, and his feet and legs were extremely swollen from accumulating fluid that had no place to go. His skin was stretched painfully tight as it attempted to expand far enough to accommodate the excess fluid. His lungs were also being flooded with fluids, which meant that he was drowning in his hospital bed. Thomas was not responding to any of the diuretics or other medications meant to release the excess fluids from his body; this only put more stress on his faltering heart. He was expected to die by morning.

When I entered the hospital room and saw him, my first thought was that Thomas looked as though he would explode if stuck with a pin. While I had been called to talk with him as a psychologist—he was one of my first patients during my internship—I did not do hypnosis with him because I had not yet completed that training.

However, I already understood the power of the mind to heal the body. I believed that if Thomas could imagine or visualize his condition improving, he might experience some relief. So I asked him, "Would you be interested in learning how your mind could help your body release this excess fluid?"

"No," came his immediate response. He shifted painfully in the hospital bed, careful not to disturb the IV in his arm. "I don't believe in that sort of thing."

As Thomas and I continued talking, a Catholic priest entered his room. Calmly and with deep compassion, he offered prayers and the Eucharist to the dying man. A devout Catholic, Thomas accepted, believing that this would be his last time to receive such gifts.

Then the priest gently placed his hand on Thomas's shoulder and looked into his eyes.

"Is there anything you need to cry about?" he asked.

Thomas appeared stunned by the question, but remained silent. Soon after, the priest and I left the room.

The next morning when I came to visit Thomas, expecting him to be even closer to death, I was astonished to learn that he was out of danger. His blood pressure was nearer to normal than it had been in many years, and the swelling in his feet and legs had been greatly reduced. He was able to breathe comfortably, since the congestion in his lungs had disappeared. The nurse saw my surprise, and she told me what had happened.

Shortly after the priest and I had left the room, Thomas had begun crying, even sobbing, and he had continued crying throughout the night. As he cried, the swelling in his body began to go down. Frequent readings showed that his blood pressure was dropping into the safe zone as well. His color had improved, and his pain level had fallen significantly.

I spoke briefly with Thomas, who was in much better spirits than during our earlier conversation. We did not mention my question to him about the power of the mind to heal the body. I didn't have to ask if such a strategy could work, because it was obvious to me that it could. Thomas was busy adjusting to the fact that he was going to live a longer, healthier life than he had anticipated only hours earlier. But I realized that even if he had not been able to believe in me or my suggestion, he had believed wholeheartedly in the priest and his question.

I have never forgotten Thomas and the lesson he taught to anyone willing to take it to heart. We say that tears come from the heart. Thomas had blocked his tears from falling—perhaps he believed that "real men" don't cry or was unable to cry for another reason—but once he was able to release the fluid of his tears, his heart responded positively. Metaphorically speaking, the dam he had built around his heart opened, allowing the harmful, excess fluid to flow out so he could be healthy again.

Heartbroken Father

Martin and Alice's daughter, Cynthia, had died of cancer when she was only eighteen. She had been an artist with a promising career and life ahead of her. Her death left her parents heartbroken, especially Martin, who refused to let his wife put photographs of either Cynthia or her artwork around the house. While Alice felt this would honor their daughter's memory and celebrate her artistic talent, Martin did not want any visual reminders of her around him. In fact, he told his wife that he did not want to speak about Cynthia or even think about her. He kept his intense grief bottled up inside.

Martin had always been healthy, but soon after Cynthia's death, he began experiencing chest pain and blood pressure that was far too high. Too often, Alice had had to call an ambulance to rush him to the emergency room. She feared she would soon lose her husband as well. After yet one more trip to the ER, and admission to the hospital, Martin's doctor requested an in-hospital consultation so he could learn stress-management techniques in hopes that this would reduce his blood pressure and resolve his heart problems.

During this hospital house call, Martin looked fragile and yet extremely tense, as if consciously holding himself together for fear that if he lost control, he would crumble into pieces. He told me about his wife's desire to celebrate Cynthia's life by putting her artwork on display in their home.

"But that would be far too heartbreaking," he told me, his voice cracking as he fought to control his emotions. "I can't bear to look at her art or a picture of her. I don't even want to talk about her." Tears came to his eyes, but he remained stoic and refused to let them fall.

We humans often reveal the real reason behind an illness in the words we use to describe our feelings or the situation in which we find ourselves. Dropping common metaphors into their conversation, my patients frequently tell me about something that is bothering them, but they do not make the connection between that language and the illness or condition that brought them to me. Additionally, they do not realize that the subconscious, or the mind of the body, will often interpret their metaphors in a literal and physical way. So when Martin used the word *heartbreaking* in reference to his daughter's death, he gave me the direction to take with his hypnosis and treatment. His heart was literally breaking because of his refusal to deal with his grief.

The first thing I taught Martin was how to use hypnosis to relax. Gradually, as he learned to relax his body, muscle by muscle, head to toe, he became more open to the idea of talking about Cynthia. In one session, when he was ready, he went into trance and I helped him create a scenario in which he embraced Cynthia, and then they were able, with much love and gratitude, to say their good-byes.

As Martin continued to use self-hypnosis and relaxation techniques, he was also able to ease his grief. To his wife's relief, he soon welcomed the idea of showcasing many pieces of Cynthia's art around the house, and he even helped his wife put them on display. As later follow-up visits to his doctor revealed, his blood pressure remained under control and he no longer had to be rushed to the ER with chest pain. Both literally and metaphorically, his "heartbreak" was easing.

Feeling the Pressure

White-coat hypertension is a mind-body phenomenon in which people have high blood pressure readings only in a doctor's office or in other clinical settings. Typically already under pressure to have healthy readings for some reason, such as a physical exam required for a job, they subconsciously begin to associate the white coat or uniform of the doctor or nurse with stress. This alone raises their blood pressure, and when the nurse or doctor issues warnings about the dangers of high readings, the stress only increases. It is easy to see how the mind of the body would then come to associate high blood pressure with similar situations, until it becomes a vicious circle. I have often used hypnosis to successfully treat people for this white-coat hypertension.

For instance, Jessica was a healthy, forty-one-year-old single mother who was applying for a job with her city government. Her current salary was being stretched thin by the needs of her children, so she needed the new, better-paying job and its benefits. The application process required her to take a physical exam, however, and even though she was in good health, this made her apprehensive.

Jessica had her blood pressure taken for this employment physical twice. Both times the readings were too high. She had no history of cardiovascular disease or high blood pressure, except when physically examined for this job. Therefore, the physician granted her one more opportunity to have her blood pressure checked.

She made an appointment to see me in order to learn how to use hypnosis to keep her white-coat hypertension under control. She learned well with a few practice attempts during an hour session.

First of all, I taught her hypnosis using progressive body relaxation. Then, as I put a blood pressure cuff around her arm, she learned to put herself in a light trance to stay relaxed. Every time I pumped the bulb to increase the pressure on her arm, she used that as a signal to her body to relax more deeply. When I put the stethoscope in the crease of her elbow, that was another signal to deepen her relaxation yet again.

I also helped Jessica create imagery she could use while waiting in the doctor's office before the exam. There, she could practice imagining her body relaxing through the entire physical exam, including the time when the blood pressure cuff was placed around her arm and pumped up. She merely had to use the signals she had learned in my office to silently tell her body to remain relaxed. We expanded the range of places where she would envision this relaxing imagery to include getting in her car to drive to the clinic, and walking from the parking lot to her doctor's office. Our goal was to associate relaxation with many of the events she would experience when going to have her blood pressure measured.

In my practice, I've seen dozens of people like Jessica who have white-coat hypertension but otherwise no history of high blood pressure. For these people, the anxiety over not getting a job was enough to create the tension that was measured as high blood pressure. In other words, the thought of the high-stakes physical exam and all that depended on it generated the emotional anxiety that the body translated into high blood pressure. In fact, I've treated many people whose anxiety and fear about having high blood pressure was so obsessive that it led them to visit malls and other places with public blood pressure devices several times a day—a behavior, of course, that kept their anxiety, and their blood pressure, at stratospheric levels.

Fortunately, with hypnosis, people can learn to feel more confident and comfortable in controlling their stress-induced anxiety by means of relaxation. Relaxation is the opposite of anxiety, so anytime you combine relaxation with hypnosis, you automatically influence and neutralize the anxiety that might be contributing to your symptoms. *Please note that I am speaking about using hypnosis to reduce hypertension by reducing anxiety and stress. Individuals with essential hypertension or cardiovascular disease require medical supervision and treatment.*

What These Cases Teach Us

Stress in our lives is inevitable, whether it stems from the heartbreak of losing a child or worry over not getting a job. However, our health, fitness level, and lifestyle affect how our body and mind handle stress. When the "pressure" of life becomes too great, the body can show signs of excessive and unhealthy strain, and that's when we need to address it.

Here, again, we see that one of the major benefits of hypnosis is how it naturally restores healthy relaxation throughout our vessels, tissues, and organs.

Chapter 8

Reproductive System: Babies and Sex

With our reproductive systems we are able to create life. Mysterious and awe-inspiring, sex, pregnancy, and birth are highly invested with emotions and deeply rooted beliefs, often buried in the subconscious. Hypnotic healing is one way to uncover and resolve hidden conflicts surrounding reproduction and fertility.

We know that our reproductive systems and fertility are influenced by stress. Today's sophisticated fertility treatments can be very draining—both financially and emotionally—and when that issue is coupled with the strong desire for a child as well as the fear that treatment will not produce one, people undergoing these treatments can become quite anxious about the outcome.

Other conditions related to the reproduction system range from conception, pregnancy, labor and delivery, to male and female sexual performance.

A Fertile Belief

Several years ago, Janice contacted me by e-mail for an Internet house call. She lived far from Tucson, where I live, and so could not visit in person. She wondered if I could prepare an audio recording of a hypnosis session she could use not only to become pregnant but to carry a healthy fetus to term. As she explained, she had had two prior pregnancies resulting from fertility treatments, but both times the fetus died after several months. She wrote that she had known the exact moment each baby died—both times a heartbreaking and traumatic experience for her.

After the failed pregnancies, her doctors recommended two options for Janice: either a hysterectomy followed by adoption of a baby, or a course of drugs she would have to take for a year before trying to become pregnant again. They warned her that the drugs would have strong, unpleasant side effects and could be toxic in other ways. Not satisfied with either of these options, Janice decided to see if hypnosis could help first. Her husband was supportive of any option she decided to choose.

I had never met Janice in person (and never would), but her story touched my heart. I could not ignore her plea for help. So after I agreed to create an audio recording for her, I spent three months researching fertility issues and ways the mind-body connection can affect reproduction. Janice and I e-mailed frequently so I could learn more about her experience, which would help me tailor the recording to her specific needs. She wrote about how traumatic it had been to lose two babies after going through difficult fertility treatments. She feared undergoing the drug treatment recommended by her doctors, as well as having to wait a year before attempting to get pregnant again. And neither did she want to have a hysterectomy, which would leave adoption as her only recourse for having a child. Even worse, her friends, whom she had counted on for support, did not offer much comfort after her miscarriages, which only increased her sadness. (I've heard similar stories from other women after a miscarriage or even an abortion. Their family, friends, or another network they had depended on for support, did not or could not acknowledge the grief caused by the loss of an unborn child.) Janice wrote that the one bright spot in this heartbreaking situation was the undying support of her husband.

About three months after Janice's first e-mail, I had created an audio recording of a hypnosis session for her. It focused primarily on instilling confidence and belief in her body's ability to perform as it was designed to perform as a woman and a mother. Instead of dealing with "issues of fertility" related to medication or surgical procedures, I was careful to put most of the emphasis on comforting her soul and her mind. My audiotape included affirmations cultivating her belief in her ability to experience a successful conception, a healthy, full-term pregnancy, and a comfortable delivery of a robust baby. In addition, I recommended that she imagine herself maintaining a healthy diet and exercise program during the pregnancy, with plenty of good sleep as the baby grew to a healthy size in her womb. Finally, I incorporated suggestions about how she could imagine herself shielded from the negative words and ideas of others who were encouraging hysterectomy and adoption, or medication. This also included protecting her from the negative effects of anyone expressing worry during her forthcoming pregnancy. In its essence, I focused the recorded session on reducing all the stresses she had described to me surrounding her fertility, pregnancies, and her worries that she might never become a mother.

When I mailed the CD to her, I asked her to use it daily and allow herself to become immersed in the belief of what she wanted and to picture in detail that it had already happened.

About a year later, a beautiful bouquet of fragrant star lilies was delivered to my office. I had no idea who had sent it. The card carried a lovely note of thanks from Janice. Attached to it was a photograph of a beautiful baby boy, with *Sammy* written on the back.

Since then, I've enjoyed working with other women who have used hypnosis to enhance their fertility and allow pregnancy and childbirth to be happy, comfortable experiences for them.

Where Do You Put Your Faith?

A physician at a local hospital called me to do a consultation on another physician's wife, Teri, thirty-one, to rule out the possibility of "drug-seeking behavior." (That is, one of the consulting doctors felt that she might be repeatedly complaining of pain in order to get narcotic pain medicine.) She had made numerous visits to the emergency department for abdominal pain. I made a hospital house call to meet with her.

As Teri told me, she had struggled for many years with severe pain resulting from fibroids, which are common and benign tumors of the uterus.

"The women in my family have always had fibroids," she said, "and doctors have told me I have a ton of them. They really do cause me a lot of pain."

A flash of deep sadness crossed her face, and I suspected that her pain was not only physical.

"My husband and I have been trying to have a baby for a long time," she continued. "But no luck. Probably because of the fibroids." Her husband, a neurosurgical resident, was immersed in the world of conventional medicine and had little familiarity with mind-body therapies.

Teri had undergone several rounds of fertility treatment, which put a strain on her marriage and the family budget, but she had never conceived as a result of the treatments. Finally, she was told that the only solution was to have a hysterectomy—removing her uterus would also eliminate the fibroids—and then adopt children. She was not yet ready to accept this verdict.

As we spoke, it became clear to me that Teri was not in the hospital with severe pain for drug-seeking behavior, as her admitting physician had suspected. Instead, she was dealing with an emotionally painful situation as she attempted to come to terms with the notion that she might never have children of her own and that the only way to stop the physical pain was through major surgery.

"There might be another way," I suggested. "I'm a psychologist who specializes in clinical hypnosis. Would you like to talk about how hypnosis might help you?"

She considered her answer for a few moments, and then said, "Yes. Everyone keeps telling me to just cut out the fibroids. But I can't do that. I'm still young enough to have kids of my own. Tell me more."

I explained how the power of the mind affects the body, usually in a subconscious way so that we do not realize what is happening. However, with clinical hypnosis it is also possible and often easy to consciously control our thoughts about a certain subject to influence our mind-body in a positive way.

"It's possible that using self-hypnosis can improve your fertility and help you get pregnant," I said. "And hypnosis can also help you manage pain, so you don't have to be at the mercy of emergency departments and analgesic medications."

"Yes, I want to learn," she said.

She discussed this with her husband and they came to my office the next week. I taught them both how to put themselves in trance and do self-hypnosis. They were surprised at how simple it was and how relaxed they felt, after months of tension over dealing with fertility issues. However, they still faced the dilemma of the medical option being offered to them: hysterectomy and adoption.

Then, point blank, I asked them, "Where do you want to put your faith? In the power of your minds to enhance fertility, or the advice about hysterectomy?"

This was not a new question for them. For two years they had had no success with fertility procedures, and they were tired of "experts" informing them that the chances of a successful pregnancy were slim to none. Teri was also ready to be done with the fibroids and the pain they caused. In short, they were ready to trust in the power of their own minds and to maintain a positive belief in having their own children.

Every day for several months, they used hypnosis to reaffirm their belief in a successful conception and pregnancy that would produce a healthy baby. They consciously reduced their anxiety and stress to improve the chances for conception, and simply to enjoy life more. They chose to see Teri's body as healthy and perfect so that her true nature could express itself in a successful pregnancy. When she felt ready, she used in vitro fertilization to become pregnant. Their prayers were doubly answered when she gave birth to healthy twins. After the births, she elected to have a hysterectomy to remedy the uterine fibroid condition.

The Memory of a Cherished Meal

Many pregnant women experience some nausea; usually it is neither severe nor long-lasting. Yet some pregnant women experience extreme, persistent nausea and vomiting that can lead to dehydration as well as malnutrition for both mother and baby. This condition is called *hyperemesis gravidarum*. Hypnosis has long been recognized as a helpful tool for alleviating this condition, as well as normal morning sickness.

I made a hospital house call to a young, expectant mother named Barbara with hyperemesis gravidarum. She had been hospitalized so she could receive intravenous nourishment and medicine for nausea. Well into her second trimester, she had spent most of her pregnancy nauseated and vomiting, and was losing instead of gaining weight. Exhausted by her ordeal, Barbara was also feeling very discouraged. Her doctors believed her condition was putting both her and the baby in jeopardy, so they had asked me to teach her how to use hypnosis to overcome the nausea (this same technique is also helpful for people with nausea caused by chemotherapy).

"Are you sure this will work?" she asked as she began to cry. "I'm so worried about the baby. And I'm so tired of not being able to keep anything down. I'm almost afraid to eat anything."

"Let's see how your tummy responds," I assured her. "Hypnosis is very easy for most people to learn. First, I'll show you how to go into trance, which you'll be able to use any time on your own."

Already in a hospital bed, she used her pillows to prop herself into a more comfortable position.

Barbara was an excellent subject for hypnosis and learned quickly how to go into trance. I then provided an experience with guided imagery by helping her use her imagination to visualize her digestive tract remaining calm, relaxed, and comfortable for the remainder of her pregnancy. We next worked on improving her appetite.

"When was a time in your life you felt happiest?" I asked.

"That was my honeymoon on Maui," she replied quickly, as a dreamy smile of remembrance swept over her face. "We stayed in the honeymoon suite at this luxurious hotel."

"During your honeymoon, were there any moments involving food when you were happy?"

"One night we had this lovely dinner at the hotel," she said. "It was one of the most delicious and romantic dinners of my life."

"That sounds like a wonderful dinner! Now use your imagination to take yourself back to that time and that dinner. Put yourself in the hotel restaurant on Maui, right across from your husband. Tell me about the food on your plate."

Barbara began by describing a table by the window with the finest ocean view. Two yellow taper candles flickered romantically. Everything on the menu sounded so delicious, she said, it was hard to make her choices. But she did, and she remembered it all—from the crab-cake appetizers to the almond-crusted halibut fillet, and then on to chocolate volcano for two. I asked her to concentrate on the flavors and fragrances of the meal so she could reexperience it all in her imagination. She had been nauseous for so long that part of her was ready to welcome reliving this romantic dinner.

As she continued reminiscing about the special meal, I suggested to her that her body responds to everything she puts into her mind.

"Your subconscious, or your mind-body, accepts the ideas you entertain in your mind," I explained. "So at any time, you can purposely create the same state of happiness you felt during this dinner. Just as you are doing now, you can take yourself back to that honeymoon dinner with your husband any time you wish, and then consciously use those same pleasant feelings in the present. Your body will respond accordingly.

"You can use this technique to improve your appetite now and for the remainder of your pregnancy," I continued, "and be free of all nausea."

Barbara had also been frightened by the negative prospects and worries over her condition expressed by her family and the medical staff, so we spent a few minutes also creating more confidence and happiness to replace the fear.

Within a few days, Barbara's nausea was well under control, and she was released from the hospital. She was once again able to enjoy eating so that she and the baby gained a healthy amount of weight. Her pregnancy continued with no further complications, and she later delivered a healthy baby.

Sometimes hyperemesis gravidarum is the result of underlying anxieties about changes that will occur when a baby enters the family. These can also be addressed in the same way as Barbara's situation: by asking the mind of the body to simply reveal information in a way that will be useful. When hypnosis reveals any hidden reasons for worry, such as fear of becoming a mother and how this will affect her life, they can then be addressed consciously. A person can also recall times of feeling confident, relaxed, and comfortable, and then apply those to the current situation to neutralize or redirect the anxiety. The body will make the connection.

No Pills Necessary

Television programs are now flooded with commercials for erectile dysfunction remedies, and e-mail in-boxes and spam folders overflow with sales pitches for pills that will "enhance your manhood." Perhaps this abundance of products and information (or, often on the Internet, misinformation) reflects the level of anxiety that many men feel about ED. Yet in my practice, hypnosis has often helped men overcome this distressing condition without drugs.

One of these patients, John, had undergone a prostatectomy recently. One of the side effects of this surgery can be impotence or difficulty in achieving an erection. While his surgeon had used the "nerve-sparing" technique, designed to leave intact the nerves that allow for an erection, the surgery was not successful in that regard. John scheduled a visit to my office after being referred to me by his family doctor and his urologist. He told me that on occasion he would awaken with a nocturnal erection, so he believed it was possible for him to achieve erection at other times. However, he confided that even prior to his surgery he had been having problems achieving an erection.

John was a teacher of anatomy and physiology, so he was well-versed in the intricate details of the human body. When he came to my office, he explained that he wanted to offer to his own mind-body the precise information it would need to enable him to have erections again. He provided all the correct anatomical information to me, and I wove it into a session of hypnosis. While he was in trance, we reviewed the physical conditions that cause an erection: the tissues of the penis become engorged with blood so that it becomes turgid and stiff. He could use this imagery as part of remembering what it feels like to have a strong, healthy erection, and I recorded this session so he could practice later at home. (Since then, I have provided many people seeking audio house calls with a recording on addressing erectile dysfunction.)

Even though John wanted exact, anatomically correct descriptions for suggestions during his trancework, I normally prefer imaginatively focusing on the outcome desired, even in cartoon-like fashion, rather than getting hung up on or obsessive about anatomical details. I would rather leave it to the subconscious, as it does this work best. However, the level of detail was appropriate for John, since it was his profession and his specific request.

Sometimes impotence stems from a physical problem related to medical conditions such as diabetes, chronic pain, or a post-surgical side effect, as we believed John had experienced. Anxiety over sexual performance or any other worry can also lead to an inability to have and sustain an erection. Guilt can produce the same effect. This has been the case with some of my patients, the usual cause being guilt over having been unfaithful.

John returned a week later, disappointed that the technique had not worked for him, despite having practiced hypnosis with the recording regularly.

"Would you be willing to ask your subconscious about this problem?" I asked, and continued to explain how the psychodynamic approach goes beyond addressing just the symptoms and looks for the underlying cause or origin for the symptoms.

"I'll try just about anything now," he said.

John went into a light level of trance and learned how to produce ideomotor finger signals for *yes* and *no*. Then I asked his mind-body, "Is there any reason why your body will not allow you to produce an erection?"

John's *yes* finger lifted immediately, even though he could not consciously recall any reason. After several more questions that brought us no closer to an answer, I asked, "Would it be all right for your mind-body to show you the obstacle to your having an erection?"

He looked uneasy and said, "Yes." Still in a light trance and looking uncomfortable, he said, "I was unfaithful to my wife," and began to cry. "I was on a business trip and met this woman. We had sex. Just that one time. I've never cheated before or since."

"When did your problems with having an erection begin?"

"A couple months after that trip, there were occasions when I couldn't perform at all. It's been two years since then and I've gone through prostate cancer and a prostatectomy and now I feel helpless."

He also confided that he wondered if his prostate cancer might have been a punishment for his infidelity. I explained how his guilt had grown over time until it interfered with his ability to become erect. That information then filtered into his conscious awareness. As we concluded the trancework, I asked, "Would it be all right for your mind-body to let you consciously manage your emotions to overcome the obstacle of your guilt?"

His *yes* finger lifted again.

He soon decided to talk with his parish priest and was able to absolve himself of the guilt surrounding his lapse in faithfulness. His ability to have and sustain an erection returned.

What These Cases Teach Us

A recurring theme in most of these cases is how stress and strong emotions are translated and expressed through the physical body. The physical expression of symptoms may or may not be in one's conscious awareness. By using hypnosis, we can access the mind-body connection (the subconscious) and receive insight about its way or manner of "thinking" and dealing with these emotional energies. Sometimes, a symptomatic approach is all that is needed. But if results are not forthcoming, then a psychodynamic approach is worth exploring. In either case, we still see the benefit of the relaxation response, which is inherent in the hypnotic process.

Chapter 9

Immune System: Always on Guard

Each of our bodies requires a constellation of intricate responses to protect itself from outside intruders, such as viruses and other pathogens, that cause illness. This is our immune system. In simple terms, the immune system attacks anything introduced into the body that it recognizes as foreign or not-our-body, and it usually works extremely well. Sometimes, as in the case of organ transplants, the immune system must be suppressed, usually with powerful drugs, to allow the body to accept the foreign organ. However, the immune system can also overprotect and attack the body itself, creating autoimmune diseases such as lupus, multiple sclerosis, and rheumatoid arthritis. This chapter describes how focusing the power of the mind through hypnosis can affect the immune system, including using hypnosis after a diagnosis of cancer. The new science of psychoneuroimmunology, which has its roots in ancient healing methods like hypnosis, is devoted to exploring how the mind-body connection influences immune responses.

House Call at My Home: A Suit of Armor

My first wife, Jody, was diagnosed with scleroderma in 1984. This is a hideous autoimmune disease in which first the skin and then the internal organs harden; this can cause intense pain and disfigurement. The original prognosis from her specialists was perhaps two more years of life. However, with the help of natural therapies and hypnosis, she lived until 1996, pain-free for all but a couple of weeks, despite being greatly disfigured by the disease.

Jody first knew something was wrong as she flew back to her hometown for her grandmother's birthday. Just as she left the plane, her hands suddenly became extremely cold and painful, as if she were holding them in ice water. This was her first episode of Raynaud's phenomenon, in which the arteries spasm and restrict blood flow. The symptoms were severe enough that her parents drove her to the hospital. In the emergency department, the doctors had to cut off her wedding ring due to the swelling, and they prescribed medication. Over the next few months, she began to develop lesions on her fingertips, which turned out to be calcium deposits; this led our doctor to suspect that her condition was scleroderma. He referred her to a rheumatologist, who confirmed those suspicions. Jody was stunned: Years before, she had seen a person with scleroderma, one of my fellow graduate students, who was disfigured by the disease and died shortly after we had graduated.

Scleroderma is an autoimmune disease, meaning that the healthy immune system, which normally protects us against disease, becomes overactive and aggressive against our own body. But scleroderma is indeed frightening: Scar tissue that mysteriously builds up throughout the body hardens the skin and internal organs. Jody's rheumatologist prescribed strong medication that would suppress her immune system, but warned that she would probably die within two years.

The initial medications were very powerful, and Jody experienced many negative side effects, so she quit taking them. Fortunately, she chose to follow a more natural course of healing, so over the next four to five years we explored many therapies and treatments for scleroderma. She also used hypnosis in several ways. She would imagine that her hands were covered by cozy mittens, which warmed them and overcame the Raynaud's symptoms. She also controlled her pain and discomfort through hypnosis, so she did not have to use pain medications.

Jody and I continued to enjoy our life together and maintain a positive outlook. As we explored different natural and nontoxic remedies, we found a physician who specialized in homeopathy, in which extremely diluted natural substances are used for treatment of illness. When this doctor met with Jody for the first time, he looked her in the eye and asked, "Why do you need this suit of armor?" This was an excellent metaphor for the way scleroderma affects the body, although Jody had no answer for him.

By 1990, Jody's ability to walk and use her legs had diminished to the point where she had to rely on a wheelchair much of the time. This is not typical for scleroderma, and neurologists and other specialists could not explain it, even after exhaustive testing. I asked her if she would be willing to use hypnosis to explore why her body might be causing the difficulty with her legs. She was reluctant, but willing to proceed. During the session, we established ideomotor signals: one finger would lift involuntarily for *yes,* another for *no,* and a third for *I don't know* or *I'm not ready to know.* Jody was an excellent hypnotic subject.

"Is there a part of you that knows why your legs have difficulty moving?" I asked her. Her *yes* finger lifted, so I continued.

"Would it be all right for that part of you to share this information about why your legs have difficulty moving?"

Her *no* finger lifted strongly.

More gently, I asked, "Would it be all right for a part of you to let you know why your legs are having this problem in a way that you could handle easily?"

Her *I'm not ready to know* finger now twitched. She could offer no further information, but her *yes* finger responded positively when I asked, "Would it be all right for your mind-body to find a way for you to have this information so that you can experience healing?"

About two hours later, she began crying and became hysterical, which was unlike her. As I held my wife, I reminded her that everything was going to be fine and asked what was happening. She would only repeat, "It can't be true! I don't believe it! It must be a lie!"

I then offered this suggestion: "There is a part of you that will let you see this information from a distance so you can talk about it and remain comfortably in control." Over the next several minutes, she began to calm down and told me she was having absolutely horrible thoughts about her most beloved grandfather. She refused to tell me what the thoughts were, saying only that she could not believe she could have such thoughts. Throughout the thirty years of our marriage, I had only heard how wonderful her grandfather was, how he had bought her and her sister a pony, and was one of her childhood heroes. He had passed away before 1960, so we could not talk with him now.

I called Jody's older sister, Carole, who responded to my mention of their grandfather with, "That bastard!" She went on to tell me that when Jody was eight years old, she had told their mother and father that their grandfather was "doing things." Carole also said that they had discovered he was "doing things" to one of her playmates in the neighborhood as well.

Carole explained that the molestation occurred when the grandparents stayed overnight. Grandmother slept with Carole, and in the same room Grandfather slept with Jody. When he got an erection during the night, he would put it between Jody's thighs and move it back and forth. When she finally told her parents about this, Grandfather was banned from spending the night. However, this was 1952, when incest was rarely discussed openly.

When hypnosis brought these deeply buried memories to light for Jody, she thought she must be going crazy. She could not believe that her grandfather would have done such a thing. However, when her mother and sister confirmed it, Jody accepted it as the truth. Yet even with this confirmation, she would not discuss it with me. For several months, our daughter, Elise, and I encouraged her to see a counselor or therapist to rid her psyche of these disturbing thoughts. She finally relented and began seeing a compassionate, gentle therapist named Adolfo Quezada. Over the next couple of years, Jody saw him once or twice a month for counseling, but she never discussed it with me.

When Elise got married in 1996, Jody was able to walk down the aisle without a walker or wheelchair; she required only a cane. Two months later, she told me she was afraid of losing her dignity due to the scleroderma and was ready to make her transition. By this time, her body was severely disfigured, and her appearance had changed dramatically. Some of her fingers had shriveled so much that it looked as though they had been amputated. On Christmas night, Jody died quietly at home, in Elise's and my arms.

Jody's rheumatologist originally said that she would live for only two years after her diagnosis. Instead, she lived for more than twelve. The disease progressed much more slowly than any predictions indicated. For a short time, she had used the medication prescribed by another rheumatologist she had learned to trust, but when it caused extensive sores in her mouth, which she could not eradicate with the power of her mind, she threw them in the garbage. She never took another drug for the scleroderma.

She was able to control the Raynaud's phenomenon and to manage and endure many of the other progressive symptoms of the disease, including intense pain, by using the power of her mind. The difficulty she experienced walking was not due to the scleroderma. Once she recalled the sexual molestation during her childhood, we understood why the muscles in her thighs and quadriceps would become "frozen," as she described it, and interfere with walking. At her memorial service, I asked her counselor, Adolfo, if Jody had spoken about the molestation. He looked at me and said, "She never mentioned it."

As much as she trusted and even loved Adolfo, she had not been able to speak to him about this trauma, nor to deal with the resulting emotional fallout. Then the comment of the homeopathic doctor made sense to me: "Why do you need this suit of armor?" I also wondered if "going back" for her grandmother's birthday had triggered her first symptoms.

Many people were impressed with Jody's ability to use her mind to manage and deal with the terrible symptoms of scleroderma, as well as to prolong her life until she saw her daughter married. Scleroderma is an autoimmune disease in which the body attacks itself; there is no genetic inheritance factor associated with it, and neither is it contagious. I believe that Jody's childhood trauma played a significant role in the progress of her disease as her mind-body attempted to protect her from further abuse by wrapping her in "armor." Her courage in managing the symptoms of this disease did not extend to dealing with possible underlying causes. Her case shows how combining both symptomatic and psychodynamic techniques helped her within the limits and boundaries she set for her life.

Torrents of Belief

I already knew Ana, a registered nurse, when she was diagnosed with lymphoma, a cancer of the lymphatic system, at age fifty. Strong and compassionate, Ana provides long-term care for patients with difficult diseases, such as the father of one of my good friends, who had Lou Gehrig's disease (ALS). I was surprised when she came to my office.

"They tell me I have lymphoma," she announced, "but I'm not going to take any of their chemotherapy. Teach me how to do self-hypnosis."

I agreed to teach her, but added, "Hypnosis is not a substitute for all the other sound, sensible medical advice you have access to, Ana. I encourage you to strongly consider working with your medical doctors as well."

Yet she was determined to follow her own course and wanted nothing to do with standard cancer treatment. I was impressed with her courage, the same kind of fierce determination with which she treated so many terminal and seriously ill patients.

"But I can't pay you," she added. "I don't have any money left."

"That's no problem at all. You've given so much compassionate care to others, now I can do the same for you," I answered.

During our first session, Ana told me she was from Tennessee and of Native American ancestry. She was very interested in using healing techniques that included imagery and "energy."

So after I had taught her basic hypnosis techniques, we practiced working with guided imagery and progressive relaxation. She easily was able to imagine a radiant light traveling through her body, delivering the healing energy. I also offered hypnotic suggestions to magnify the benefits of the food, water, and medicines that her immune system would need to restore her to health.

She returned in two weeks for her next appointment.

"How are you doing?" I asked.

"Very well, I think. Here's how I'm using my hypnosis . . ."

First a bit of explanation for nondesert dwellers: In the Southwest, many riverbeds remain bone-dry most of the year.

Called arroyos, or dry washes, these ancient pathways contain water only during or after rainstorms; when the rain is powerful enough or lasts long enough, the rushing water can become a torrent of immense energy. One of these arroyos ran near Ana's house, and she had often walked it during the dry seasons to experience the power of the desert's special beauty.

Since our first session, she had discovered a place in the arroyo where she could comfortably lie down, and she began doing her hypnosis there. She would stretch out on her back, close her eyes, and let herself ease into trance. Then she used her own personal healing imagery: She began by imagining the many centuries it had taken to carve this arroyo out of the hard desert soil. Next, she deepened her sensory experience by imagining the vast amounts of energy still present in that place from all the torrents of pounding water. Then she imagined a strong energy connection rising from the earth and into her body, and how this energy that had also created the arroyo was a creative energy now flowing through her body, too, rinsing it free and clear of any cancer cells.

"I'm quite pleased with this imagery," she told me, "and the way it merges with how I feel about nature and spirituality."

"Yes, it sounds like it's working for you," I said. "Keep it up."

Ana returned for our third and last session, but only to give me a jar of black-eyed peas she had canned herself. This was her payment to me.

I worked with Ana in 1992. She later returned to Tennessee and still remains healthy and active.

Fishing for an Appetite

Bruce had a type of bone cancer that was spreading throughout his body when his wife brought him to see me. He was receiving a heavy course of strong chemotherapy that left him severely nauseated after each treatment. He could not eat for a day or two afterward, and his weight was falling dramatically.

An architect, Bruce was analytical and methodical, as well as creative, so I approached his hypnosis the same way. He was able to convert many of the ideas I explained to him into detailed plans, much as he would go about designing the structure for a library or another building.

After learning some trance-induction methods, he learned how to detach himself from his surroundings. One of his favorite activities was fly fishing, so he quickly learned to imagine himself standing in a mountain stream, casting for trout and other fish, on a beautiful sunny day. As we practiced, I asked him if he was fly fishing at that moment, and when he was, I continued with another suggestion to his subconscious.

"Wouldn't it be interesting to discover what foods your mind-body is craving as a result of your fly fishing while you're receiving your chemotherapy?" I asked. "When you're standing in that river on a beautiful day doing something you enjoy so much, I don't know if you would be craving a slice of juicy watermelon or a hot baked potato. I don't know if you would be craving one of your favorite foods. But I do know you will have a wonderful sense of security and comfort in knowing that your mind-body is responding to your wishes to overcome any side effects of the chemotherapy."

Bruce began applying his new skill during his next chemotherapy session at the hospital. When he came to our next appointment, I noticed he did not look as gaunt and worn-out as he had the week before.

"The strangest thing is happening, Doc," he said.

"What's that?" I asked, although I had a happy suspicion about what he was going to say.

"It used to be that after chemo, I would throw up for the rest of the day and the day after. But now, even before I finish receiving all the chemo drugs, I get this craving for pizza." He laughed. "So we go home and make a homemade pizza with all my favorite ingredients."

Bruce's weight continued to improve and he never had another problem with any side effects of chemotherapy. His story illustrates a common way of addressing the side effects of nausea and vomiting associated with chemotherapy or any type of condition. That is, together, my patient and I look for the opposite of the symptom, and work to create that opposite in the imagination first, so the body can then follow suit. If the symptom is anxiety, we emphasize relaxation. If my patient feels as if a part of his or her body is on fire, as can happen with some medical conditions and treatments, we emphasize soothing, cooling images and colors. As with Bruce, the opposite of nausea and not being able to eat is having a desire to eat. When an even stronger solution is needed, we create a craving to eat, which is stronger than a desire.

The Doctor Doesn't Believe in Any of This

Dr. Ed, a scientist and engineer in his seventies, came to my office with his wife, Dolores. As soon as he sat down at the table where I first meet with my patients, he announced, "I want to tell you right off, I don't believe in any of this." He pointed to his wife and said, "I'm only here because of her. She dragged me to see Dr. Wheel, too, and I don't believe in what he does, either!" He was referring to my colleague, Andrew Weil, MD (pronounced "while").

I expect resistance from everyone, myself included, whenever talking about a new concept or altering old habits or beliefs. However, Dr. Ed's level of resistance was so high that I was not about to challenge him directly.

"That's fine," I said to him. "If your wife wants you to be here, why don't I just talk with her? I'll teach your wife to use these techniques. I'd rather do that than have you feel that you wasted your money by coming here."

They were both delighted with my suggestion. He believed he had turned the tables on his wife, who was worried about him because he had multiple myeloma cancer and was not responding to chemotherapy. She wanted to explore other approaches at the Arizona Center for Integrative Medicine in Tucson, which Dr. Andrew Weil had founded and where I am on the faculty. But as a retired engineer with an extremely analytical mind, he was not imaginatively engaged in pursuing alternative oncology treatments.

So I spoke with Dolores and asked her questions about herself as if she were my patient. I explained how hypnosis works, how she could learn it, and what she would experience. All the while, Dr. Ed sat with his arms and legs crossed in a clear statement of body language that he wanted no part of what I was saying to his wife.

When the time came for her to experience hypnosis, I invited her to sit in one of the recliners in my office. Then I said to her husband, "There won't be anything to see while we do this. You're more than welcome to sit in the other recliner while I work with Dolores."

He accepted my invitation and made himself comfortable next to her.

Even though I worked with his wife, I directed the entire session to him in ways that did not challenge his beliefs but did provide information about the research and the empirical basis for using medical hypnosis. I provided the information I wanted him to absorb so he could have the opportunity to change his beliefs, based on sound information.

During the trancework with Dolores, we used an induction method that included progressive body relaxation, and then I guided her with imagery. While she was in trance, I suggested that she was on a path that led to a gentle waterfall and described how she could stand under the water, with it falling gently upon her.

"The water is now turning into light," I continued, "and we all know that light is a form of energy. Quantum physicists believe that everything is energy, and they know that atoms are mainly open space filled with energy, rather than solid objects."

Dolores nodded, still in trance, and appeared to be enjoying her experience with the imaginary lightfall.

"Now the light falling upon you is beginning to change color, and these different colors represent different wavelengths of energy," I continued. "Each wavelength of energy is another resonance or vibration that can affect the space it occupies, as well as the solid parts of the cells, atoms, and molecules of the body." I paused for a moment, and then said, "Any illness and any cancer is a shadow, and we all know what happens when light is shined on a shadow."

Just about that time, Dr. Ed's whole body twitched. This was a myoclonic movement, which is the natural result of a body relaxing and releasing tension. This often happens just as we fall asleep.

When Dolores and I finished the trancework, I could tell that Dr. Ed was eager to tell me something. But I kept politely postponing him, explaining that it was important for me to finish talking with his wife. I then asked her more questions than I ordinarily would, which further built up his eagerness to tell me his news. I finally turned to him and asked casually, "Did you experience anything?"

Dr. Ed could hardly sit still as he explained how he had been able to visualize the electron rings, neutrons, and protons within the atoms, how the light from the waterfall traveled through space, and how the vibration of the wavelengths of light energy affected the energy within each atom. Finally, he said, "I could even see the shadows instantly disappear when the light was shined on them!"

At the end of the session, he apologized to me for being so

"difficult." He was not about to acknowledge the shift in his beliefs, but he admitted that he was glad they had come to see me and felt he had learned something. As I often do, I had recorded the session and then created a CD for him and his wife. I recommended that they could both use it on a daily basis until their mind-bodies memorized how to follow the instructions they were providing through their imaginations.

About six months later, I received a call from Dr. Ed's oncologist.

"What happened when he was in your office?" he asked.

"Nothing much," I said.

"Well, something happened because he is attributing his visit to you with the reason we can't find any cancer in his body."

I explained how Dr. Ed had been a challenging subject, but I knew he was motivated to heal and was gracious enough to allow his wife to be the focus of attention that day. I added that I had created a CD from the session and gave it to them, along with instructions for practicing hypnosis.

Just a few months after the call from the oncologist, Dr. Ed e-mailed me a kind message, explaining how grateful he was for the experience with hypnosis and how he believed that the power of his mind was instrumental in his healing from cancer. At the end of the e-mail, he had written, "Will this work for my tennis game, too?"

Dr. Ed's case demonstrates how a person's belief can be the greatest obstacle to being able to benefit from the power of the mind in the form of hypnosis. I expect resistance. It is normal. Dr. Ed's resistance was extreme in my experience, so I never challenged him. Instead, I simply offered evidence and information about empirical studies, all of which were true. Obviously, the statement that had the most effect on him was, "We all know what happens when light is shined on a shadow." That was the moment of truth for Dr. Ed, and when he learned that truth, he was able to benefit.

I Like Your Necktie

Each week, the doctors-in-training in our integrative medicine program spend an afternoon in our patient conference in order to present and discuss the cases seen that week. Many specialties are represented, including botanical medicine, homeopathy, energy healing, osteopathic medicine, physical therapy, pharmacy, mind-body medicine, nutrition, shamanism, traditional Chinese herbs and acupuncture, spirituality, and other healing techniques. At this time, Dr. Andrew Weil, founder of the Arizona Center for Integrative Medicine at the University of Arizona, always joined us.

At one patient conference, a doctor in the fellowship brought along a patient and announced to everyone that I would be working with him. This was the first time a patient had ever attended one of these meetings. Richard, a young man in his early forties, had lost his sight through an accident while making jewelry. As he explained it, he was working with molten silver, and when he added another reagent to the molten silver, the mixture accidentally splashed into his eyes, burning the corneas. He had already received three corneal transplants, but his body had rejected all of them within six months to two years following the implantations. Because of this, he was now considered ineligible for another attempt at a transplant, a state of affairs that would leave him blind for life. The doctor who brought Richard to the conference believed he could use the power of his mind to prevent his immune system from rejecting new corneas, should he have the opportunity to receive a fourth transplant. During this conference, Richard allowed me to demonstrate simple hypnosis exercises to determine his initial talent with hypnosis. He appeared to be an excellent hypnotic subject.

Due to his lack of sight, Richard had a difficult time traveling, so I made four house calls to his home. I would always call to let him know I was on my way, and when I arrived, he would come to the door and I would announce myself.

Initially, I instructed Richard in the techniques of hypnosis so he could feel comfortable going into trance or entering a day-dreamlike state of reverie in which he could turn on his imagination. Then, he or I offer hypnotic suggestions he could use for healing with words or images in his mind. I also taught him how to create involuntary ideomotor responses with his fingers, where one finger represented *yes,* another *no,* and a third *I don't know* or *I'm not ready to know.*

In the course of our trancework, I asked his mind-body, or subconscious, various questions. Sometimes, the results revealed a hidden inner conflict. For instance, every time I asked him, "Is your immune system ready to accept new corneas?" he said aloud, "Of course I'm ready," but his *no* finger lifted. His conscious and subconscious minds clearly were not in agreement. He was not aware of which fingers were lifting or twitching as he verbally answered many of the questions I asked his mind-body. I looked for clues as to how I might help him safely resolve this conflict.

He and his wife did not have children, although I noticed scattered about his house a number of books about having a baby, pregnancy, and fertility. I crafted a story while Richard was in trance about how people who cannot have biological children will adopt a child and treat it as their very own flesh and blood. Even though the child did not come from their own genetic code and cells, they raise it within the family with love and care, making no distinctions about the origins of the physical or genetic material of their child.

Then I expanded the story into how he could talk with his immune system, suggesting that new corneas are desirable for sight and that corneas he could receive would not have the same genetic makeup or DNA. Richard knew that one of the major tasks of the immune system is to protect him from invaders or intruders into his body, so during our trancework, I commended his immune system on doing an excellent job of protecting him. Then I described how new corneas would be like adopting a baby into the family and embracing it with love, nurturing, and protection.

Once again, I asked his immune system, "Would you be willing to protect the new corneas you adopt into your body and love them as your own?" Just as before, he replied aloud with "Yes," but this time, his *yes* finger quivered slightly while his *no* finger remained motionless. He was moving in the right direction.

I continued this line of reasoning for a few more minutes, then again asked, "Is your immune system ready to welcome a new member of the family, new corneas, and to love them and protect them as your very own for as long as you live?" By now, his *yes* finger was lifting more emphatically, as his *no* finger still remained motionless.

I suggested to Richard that he call his ophthalmologist and ask to be added to the cornea transplant list once more. His doctor agreed, and shortly thereafter Richard received the corneas of a young woman who had died in a motorcycle accident. Since my office was across the street from the hospital where he had the surgery, I saw him immediately afterward in the surgical recovery room to reinforce my earlier suggestions about lovingly accepting and protecting his new corneas as a member of his family of cells and tissues for as long as he lives. His *yes* finger lifted again, moving comfortably in agreement with his verbal, "Of course."

Several weeks later, I stopped by his house to see how he was doing. First, I called him to let him know I was on my way, as I had in the past. When he opened the door, before I could say a word, he said, "I like your necktie." He could see!

Richard's case is a good example of using hypnosis to very selectively suppress the immune system. We usually think of enhancing it, but in this case, partial suppression was necessary so the body would accept foreign tissue as a new member of the "family."

What These Cases Teach Us

The cases in this chapter differ from those in the other chapters because the role of stress and anxiety is not as evident. However, some of these cases illustrate how strong emotional energy may have devastating effects, particularly when there is a conflict between the conscious mind and the subconscious, or the mind of the body. What we learn from this chapter is that the power of belief is a vital ingredient for making hypnosis effective. In some of the cases, it was easy to channel belief into a positive experience, mentally and physically. In the case of Dr. Ed, we see the power of changing belief and using it. That is, it didn't matter how strongly he disbelieved or resisted believing in mind-body methods. Once his belief changed, that's all that mattered.

This chapter also involves cases of serious and often fatal illness. Some of the people integrated hypnosis along with their medical therapies, and some refused the pharmaceutical treatments. I encourage everyone to evaluate and integrate conventional allopathic medical therapies and other healing modalities that are shown to be effective.

Chapter 10

Pain: Controlling the Hurt

While we usually do everything we can to avoid pain, it does have an essential function: to alert us that something is wrong inside our bodies. When using hypnosis to deal with pain, it is important to first be sure that any underlying condition, such as infection, is dealt with and treated. I have helped many people learn to manage and release pain through hypnosis.

Going to Mt. Lemmon

Sandra first came to see me for hypnosis when she was a teenager. She suffered from severe migraines and had been taking a prescribed narcotic to deal with the intense pain. But when she decided she no longer wanted to have the migraines nor to use narcotics, her mother, Rita, brought her to learn hypnosis. She was a quick study and rapidly got control over the migraines using the power of her mind.

Some years later, Rita called me in a panic one night. I had just finished packing and was getting ready to leave for the airport to catch a late-night flight to attend a professional conference.

"Sandy's in terrible pain and you've got to see her in the hospital tonight," Rita pleaded. "She just had extensive knee surgery, and even though they're giving her injections every couple of hours to control the pain, it's not working at all. She's writhing in pain. Can you go see her?"

I promised to stop in to see Sandra on the way to the airport.

When I arrived at the hospital, Sandra's nurse explained that frequent injections of Demerol were having no effect on the pain. When I saw Sandra, she was indeed suffering as a result of her surgery the day before.

"The pain *is* bad," she said, "because I can't control the muscle spasms."

I pulled back the sheet to look at her leg. The muscles above and below her knee were in spasm and twitching furiously.

"Do you remember your hypnosis?" I asked.

Grimacing in pain, she nodded.

"That's good. Close your eyes and relax as much as you can. Can you imagine going to your favorite place?"

She nodded again, having rapidly gone into trance. "I'm going to Mount Lemmon."

In the Catalina Mountains north of Tucson, Mount Lemmon is a popular spot for hiking, a cool location high above the hot desert floor. It was also the place where Sandra had fallen and injured her knee during a hike. Nevertheless, she always felt comfortable and happy there.

"Good," I said. "Can you describe this favorite place to me? What are you experiencing through your senses in this place?"

Sandra provided an elaborate description: the cool air several thousand feet above Tucson, the dense forest and the sound of the wind in the pine trees, the crunch of gravel and twigs under her feet on the trail, and most of all the freedom she felt there, away from her everyday cares, and now away from the confining hospital setting.

"Now, simply let the muscles in your leg spasm freely," I said. "Give them all the permission they *need* to twitch and move.

"By emphasizing the word *need*," I explained, "this will allow your body to use its inner wisdom to heal. Your surgeon is well-trained, and he did a wonderful job of performing all the mechanical repairs your knee required. Now your subconscious and your body have the wisdom that will let them put everything back in its absolutely proper position so your knee will once again be flexible and strong and perfect. The muscle spasms are merely your body doing its inner work of healing and putting all the muscle fibers and tissues back into their proper place."

I could see that Sandra was following my words while continuing to imagine herself on Mount Lemmon. So I began telling her a story that Dr. Milton Erickson was famous for. He was a respected psychiatrist who specialized in medical hypnosis and was a founding member of the American Society of Clinical Hypnosis. He was a great influence on my work, particularly in learning how to communicate with the subconscious—the mind of our body—and how it literally uses pictures, words, and ideas, along with our beliefs, to express and manifest our beliefs of the moment, whether they be for comfort or distress. He showed me how, once the subconscious mind accepts an idea, it acts upon it as real, no matter how imaginatively it may be introduced. He taught many students, including me, how to use the unique logic of the subconscious, which allows anything to be possible, as you'll see by the story I told Sandra.

"A woman was brought to his office in a wheelchair from the hospital," I began. "She was in terrible pain and was not responding to the injections of Demerol. So Dr. Erickson asked her to picture a large Bengal tiger crouched in the doorway of his office. He asked her to picture that tiger very clearly, to precisely see the colors and the length of its fur, to notice the texture and color of its gums, to see its teeth, and to also notice that its hind muscles and haunches were becoming tense and quivering, as if it were about to pounce upon her."

At that moment, the woman jerked in fright, and then he immediately asked her what she was experiencing. She said she was scared. He then asked her if she felt any pain in that moment. "No, in that moment I only thought of the tiger about to pounce."

"So Dr. Erickson asked her to go back to the hospital," I continued. "She did. And he later heard that every time someone came to give her an injection of Demerol, she said, 'I don't need it. I have a tiger under my bed.'"

I said to Sandra, "Now I suggest to you that the mind of your body, your subconscious, knows what to do with every cell of your body and also with every word of the story I just told."

Sandra continued in trance. I offered the suggestion that she would have a wonderful sleep that night and for nights afterward, and that she would continue to feel better and better as she allowed her body to perform its inner work of healing after the surgery. I left her hospital room to allow her trance to transition into a peaceful sleep.

Three days later, after returning from the conference, I stopped by the hospital to see Sandra, but she was not there.

"She was doing so well, we discharged her a day early," the nurse told me. "Since your visit the other night, Sandra refused all the pain medication." The nurse went on to tell me that each time she came to give her the prescribed injection for pain, Sandra told her, "I don't need it. I'm going to Mount Lemmon now." The nurse said, "We were going to call in a psychiatrist until her mother explained that she was using her hypnosis to imagine herself on Mount Lemmon where she was pain-free. But when she was leaving us to go home, I still insisted that she take two aspirin, just to be sure she had something to make her comfortable on the trip home."

I called Sandra's house and spoke to her. She said she was

doing very well. "From the moment I thought about how the muscles spasms were performing the inner work of healing, just as you explained, I would let go of trying to control the spasms," she explained.

As Sandra's case clearly demonstrates, anxiety and pain can build on each other. However, if we have the ability to detach and reframe our beliefs about an event, we also reframe the way our body experiences that event.

An interesting note: When I saw her that night in the hospital, she was in great pain, but she was more distressed by her inability to control the muscle spasms. When she followed my suggestion to believe that the spasms were the healthy result of her body repositioning muscle fibers and tissues, she was able to let go and relax so that her body could use its own natural chemistry to produce hypnoanalgesia or hypnoanesthesia. This is the body's natural ability to lessen or remove pain simply by using the power of the mind. The story I told about Dr. Erickson and the lady with the tiger under her bed reinforced Sandra's ability to use her hypnosis to imagine being on Mount Lemmon, where she was always comfortable.

Saints and Angels

When Francisco was carrying a heavy tray of dishes, he walked into a plate-glass patio door and fell backwards. He ruptured two discs in his neck and one in his lower back. To correct the damage, he had two surgeries on his neck and two on his back. Unfortunately, the surgeries resulted in chronic pain, which he found very difficult to endure, so he came to see me for pain relief through hypnosis.

While he appeared to be a good hypnotic subject, none of the usual techniques of going into trance and then using imagery with favorite places produced good results. After several sessions, Francisco still felt a great deal of pain.

So at our next appointment, as he was as deeply into trance as he could then go—which was very light—I asked his subconscious mind, "What will let you go into a deeper level of trance where you have only comfort?"

"I want to work with the angels and saints," he whispered.

Francisco was a devout Catholic who prayed daily to his favorite saints and believed in their protection, along with that of the angels.

With this guidance from his subconscious, I was able to help Francisco imagine the loving saints and angels of his faith coming to relieve his pain. He could clearly envision them surrounding him, blessing him, and acknowledging that they heard his prayers.

With that session, he became able to reach a deeper level of trance on his own, where he felt peaceful and safe. He feels no pain during these times, and afterwards his pain is much reduced.

Francisco is a good example of how people can use very personal images and beliefs during hypnosis to find the imagery and ideas that work best for them.

Fly Like an Eagle

Alberta's case is similar to Francisco's above. An older woman, Alberta fractured her pubic bone and pelvis in a fall; her bladder was also injured, which required surgical repairs. Afterward, the displacement of the pubic bones meant that she felt great pain upon any kind of movement. When she came to me for hypnosis, she told me of her love for nature. Like Francisco's saints and angels, nature became the path to Alberta's pain relief.

While she was going into trance, I suggested she could feel free to become any animal she wanted to be. When she came out of trance, she explained how, at first, she became an eagle and enjoyed the freedom of flying high over the desert canyons. But then she came back to earth and discovered further significant pain relief in imagining herself to be a tall, old, sturdy Ponderosa pine, rooted firmly in Mother Earth.

So whenever Alberta needs relief from pain now, she reflects on the qualities of being a free-flying eagle and a sturdy pine that has withstood many storms. Her pain level typically falls from seven out of ten to a one out of ten. Applying the strengths and glories of Mother Nature to her own mind-body nature allows Alberta to manage her pain very effectively.

Pain with a Purpose

Sally is a young and gifted stained-glass artist and welder who sustained an inguinal groin hernia (a tear in the lining of the abdomen near the groin) on the job. She had surgery to correct it, but afterward remained in chronic pain. Since she had a history of substance abuse, her doctors at first dismissed her complaints of pain as possible drug-seeking behavior.

When she came to see me, she was adamant that her substance abuse was in the past and she had no desire to become addicted again. She explained that her pain was very real and was not being relieved by the medications she had been prescribed.

I was puzzled when this highly motivated woman, who was an excellent hypnotic subject, could achieve no relief from her pain through hypnosis. In seven or eight sessions we covered all the usual techniques as well as every psychological, symptomatic, and psychodynamic angle I could think of using. Sally did her best, but nothing changed. Rarely had I seen such a stubborn case in all my years of practice.

I began to believe that there was some organic cause for her pain, perhaps resulting from the hernia surgery. I contacted her insurance company and explained the situation, along with a possible solution. "Would you authorize payment for exploratory surgery for her?" I asked.

The insurance representative laughed and said, "In this day and age, there are no exploratory surgeries."

"Perhaps you'll make an exception in Sally's case," I replied. "She's disabled with chronic pain resulting from an on-the-job injury, which means you could very well be required to pay her $1,200 in monthly disability payments for the rest of her life."

That prospect changed the representative's mind, and she authorized payment for the operation.

I asked three of my colleagues—Timothy Putty, a neurosurgeon; Dr. Jame Herde, a vascular surgeon; and Dr. Randall Prust, Sally's pain specialist and anesthesiologist—to perform Sally's surgery. They allowed me to stand in and observe—and they discovered a suture that had been placed directly across one of the nerves in Sally's groin. They removed it, and her pain disappeared, allowing her to return to her welding job.

This is one of the rare instances I've seen in which pain was not relieved with hypnosis. However, the failure of hypnosis in a highly motivated and excellent hypnotic subject suggested that the pain was still serving a vital purpose.

Above the Pain

Emily was a passenger in her employer's car when suddenly he began speeding down busy city streets. Unbeknownst to her then, he was a drug dealer, and he believed they were being followed, so he tried to elude their pursuer. After several terrifying minutes, his car hit another car head-on and was then struck by two more vehicles. Her employer was killed instantly, but Emily, twenty-four at the time, survived with internal injuries and a horrific number of fractures: skull, several vertebrae in her neck and back, both collarbones and shoulders, both upper and lower arms, several fingers and ribs, and her legs. She also had a brain injury, which left her in a coma for about four months.

Three years later, she was sent to my office. Walking and moving were still difficult for her because of all the once-broken bones—she joked that she could certainly tell when the weather was about to change!—but her mind was clear and sound. She had a positive outlook. However, her doctors had referred her to me because they were concerned that she had developed a tolerance to the heavy narcotics she had been taking to relieve her pain ever since coming out of her coma.

Agreeable to learning hypnosis for pain control, Emily easily went into trance. But she did not follow the typical hypnotic pattern. Instead, she spontaneously regressed to the time of her coma. She was able to talk with me, so I asked her what she was experiencing.

For many minutes, she talked about the doctors who treated her, some of whom she liked; others she despised. She recalled how her primary-care doctor would come into her room, followed by an entourage of residents. She hated these visits: The doctor would talk about "this twenty-something Caucasian woman" as he pulled the sheet and blanket off her body, then point out her injuries and other areas of her body. He would then turn and leave the room, his entourage following, without even bothering to cover her naked body. She remembered being cold and ashamed every time he displayed her in this fashion, as if she were a specimen to be studied instead of a badly injured human being. This was the doctor she despised.

But she also remembered one of the residents with great fondness and respect. He was often the last of the entourage to leave her room, and he took the time to rearrange her bed linens and cover her. He usually said a few kind words to her. Emily also recalled family members, including her aunts and uncles, who had come to visit, along with her parents. Some of her visitors brought gifts.

Still in trance, Emily explained to me that while she was comatose, she viewed the events in her hospital room from a vantage point near the ceiling. Floating up there, she said, she could see her body and everything else below her in the room.

For her next visit, I asked Emily to bring her mother along to confirm her story. Sure enough, her mother was able to verify the details about Emily's visitors, including who they were, the gifts they brought, and even what some of them wore.

I asked Emily what finally brought her out of the coma.

"It was the young resident who was always so kind to me," she said. "He was standing near my bed one day with another resident, and he said, 'I think she's going to make it.' I woke up right then, back in my body—but in such pain I could hardly stand it."

As a clinical psychologist who uses medical hypnosis, it was fascinating for me to hear Emily's story. She was "present" in her hospital room, even though she was in a coma, and able to hear and see whatever was going on around her. Despite being unconscious, some part of her was actively aware and paying attention—and just hearing those few positive words from a kind person who cared about her was enough to bring her out of the coma. Some people believe that those in a coma have not yet decided whether to return to their body or continue on. Her mother's corroboration of some of the details suggests credible but unexplainable trance memory. Emily's story, and others I have heard, causes me to believe that when people are comatose, they can still have awareness and be able to hear and "see" everything that happens in their environment. Although limited, it is my experience that individuals who have been in coma or have had near-death experiences often are excellent hypnotic subjects and have great talent for using self-hypnosis. Emily was able to use hypnosis to manage pain to wean herself off the narcotic medication and continue healing.

Two-Year Headache

On the job as a repair technician of automatic transmissions, Doug, then forty-eight, was carrying a heavy transmission when he fell backward, injuring his back and hitting his head. The back injury required surgery, which his doctors declared successful. Yet two years later, Doug still suffered from ongoing pain in both his lower back and his head. While his backache was sporadic, the pain in his head was continuous and intense.

"When did you first notice the headache?" I asked while taking his medical history.

"Immediately after my back surgery," he said. "That's all I know."

During two sessions, I guided Doug in doing different forms of hypnotic pain relief, but nothing worked. The pain in his head remained intense.

So I looked into his medical records and found that, prior to surgery, Doug had received a diagnostic procedure called a myelogram, in which some spinal fluid is removed from the spinal canal and replaced with a dye. The patient is placed on a table that can be tilted so that the dye flows to the area where the nerves are being imaged to examine them for damage. This could offer some clues to the source of Doug's two-year headache.

When I asked Doug about the myelogram, he recalled that the hospital's electrical power had gone out while he was in the middle of the test, just when the table was positioned so that his head was lower than the rest of his body. The technician performing the test became noticeably frightened; Doug recalled hearing him say that if he could not raise Doug's head, all the dye would flow into his brain. In the few moments before the emergency power came on, he frantically tried to readjust the table to raise Doug's head. After he tilted the table, he tapped and even pounded on the top of Doug's head to reposition the dye lower in his spine. Then the power came back on, and the myelogram was completed. The next week, Doug had spinal surgery, which his doctors pronounced a success. None of this explained the continuing headache, however.

So I guided Doug into trance and suggested, "Go back to where the headache began." I anticipated that he would regress to the time of the myelogram, but instead he began describing the scene in the operating room.

"I'm lying on my side on the operating table," he recalled, "and I can hear the doctors talking, even though I'm already under from the anesthetic. One of them was telling everyone about the power going off during my myelogram the week before and how the technician had to pound on my head to make sure the dye wouldn't flow into my brain."

He smiled. "Then my surgeon joked, 'This poor guy is going to have a headache for the next two years.'"

There was the answer! While under anesthesia, Doug's subconscious had taken the surgeon's statement literally and created the headache that had not gone away since. Unfortunately, even that conscious realization did not relieve Doug's headache.

But the second anniversary of his back surgery was only four months away. On that exact day, his headache disappeared, as his subconscious finally released him from the grip of his surgeon's literally prophetic words.

However, Doug's back pain continued, even though his surgeons believed the repair to his spine to be completely successful. Before his injury, he had been able to rebuild up to ten transmissions a day—he was a master of this work and well-known for it—but now he could hardly complete even one repair before becoming disabled by the pain. I asked Doug if I could watch him rebuild an automatic transmission in the workshop at his home, and I made a house call. During my college years, I worked as a mechanic, so I was familiar with automotive repair. I was curious to see Doug at work. Perhaps I would discover a clue to his back pain.

I was impressed and amazed at how efficiently he had designed his shop and workbench, with all his tools in precise positions, precisely laid out for transmission rebuilding. He had an automatic transmission totally disassembled, all the parts soaking in a bucket full of cleaning solvent. As I watched, he pulled out all the pieces one by one and began reassembling the transmission. Halfway through, he began to hold his lower back and said he had to go inside and lie down because of the pain.

As I had observed Doug at work, I noticed something interesting: Every time his right hand reached for a tool, his left hand would push it out of the way and pick up the tool. I asked Doug if he was right- or left-handed, and he confirmed that he was right-handed. So I showed him how his left hand took over for the right, something he did not realize was happening.

I referred Doug to a neuropsychologist colleague for tests, which confirmed that Doug had suffered damage to the area of his brain that dealt with spatial relationships and eye-hand coordination. He had hit his head on the concrete floor at work when he fell, but concern over his spinal injury had overshadowed the fact that he had also suffered a mildly traumatic brain injury. This injury caused his left hand to compensate for his right hand, which could no longer distinguish size or even the right tool. The neuropsychologist designed some cognitive exercises Doug used to strengthen the damaged area of his brain, and over time he was able to retrain his right hand to work correctly. His back pain diminished greatly.

His postsurgery back pain had not resulted from any problem with the surgery, as his doctors correctly had maintained. Instead, it was a subconscious reaction to the frustration he felt in not being able to perform his job as masterfully as he once had. Although hypnosis was not the complete answer to Doug's headache and back pain, it did lead us in useful directions. And with greater insight into his pain, Doug was able to use hypnosis to better manage his discomfort.

Common Headaches

Headaches are common and have a number of sources. They are also complex physical conditions that run the gamut from vascular headaches, like migraines, resulting from blood vessel problems, to those produced by muscle tension, to those caused by mechanical problems with posture and the neck and shoulders, to those caused by injury. Hypnosis is a helpful remedy for all kinds of headaches, from acute pain that comes on suddenly then stops, to chronic pain that continues or persists over time.

Some standard hypnotic methods work well to relieve headaches. One focuses on relaxation of the head, face, jaw, neck, shoulders, and upper body. This includes suggestions to allow the blood vessels in the hands and feet to enlarge and dilate, which allows more circulation in the hands, warming them. As you continue to relax more deeply, your hands become warmer and warmer, which can ease a headache, even a migraine.

In addition, as you relax and perhaps imagine yourself in a peaceful, favorite place, your brain will release peptides we call endorphins, or natural brain chemicals, that generate pleasure sensations in the body. In fact, endorphins resemble morphine in their chemical makeup. You may have felt the results of your body's automatic endorphin production during hard exercise or exertion, but with the deep relaxation available through hypnosis, you can create the same feelings on purpose.

If you have a headache and want to use hypnosis for yourself, start with muscle relaxation. Consciously relax the muscles of your head and face, then your neck and shoulders, and then relax more. You can add imagery or visualization that will "take" you to another location that is peaceful and restorative for you. Use your senses to re-create that location in your mind—a beach, a meadow, or any place where you can experience peace all around you—and let your cares float away. Often, your headache will float away, too.

If you have frequent headaches, it is worth asking your subconscious what the headache represents. As you relax deeply, you can silently ask yourself, "Who's the pain in the neck?" or "What's making me so uptight?" If an answer comes to mind, you can address it. If it contributes to your headaches, addressing it will also help relieve the headaches.

Painless Dentistry

Another type of acute pain can occur in the dentist's office. When I first learned about hypnosis as a teenager, I used it to overcome my phobia of needles. But I still did not like the idea of injections in my mouth, so I quickly translated this ability into creating my own anesthesia for dental procedures.

Shortly after I moved to Tucson forty years ago, I developed a toothache and went to see a kindly, elderly dentist. He informed me that I needed a root canal, and I said I wouldn't need any anesthetic. I knew I would do anything to avoid an injection, and I also knew that hypnosis would allow me to be comfortable during the procedure. However, the dentist insisted on the injection, warning me that a root canal is a painful procedure. I remained equally insistent. He eventually gave in and said, "I'll have the syringe right here, and you tell me the moment you want me to give it to you."

As he began working on my mouth, I imagined that I was somewhere else, enjoying some of the new sites and scenery I had discovered in my new home, the Sonoran Desert, where Tucson is located. I felt no distress and no discomfort at all as the root canal proceeded, yet I noticed that the dentist was constantly saying things like, "This must be killing you! How can you stand it?" Or "Are you ready for me to give you the Novocaine now?" I would shake my head, and he would continue. The stress must have been affecting him because I noticed that he would tremble or perspire and have to leave the room for a time. Meanwhile, I continued my imaginary trip through the beautiful desert and never once felt any pain.

I continued to see this dentist for several more years. I always refused the Novocaine, and he always told me how much pain I would experience, encouraging me to take the injections. One day I was scheduled for work on a molar, and when I entered the waiting room, two members of his staff took me aside and pleaded with me to take the injections.

"But I don't need it," I explained. "And I don't want it."

"Use the Novocaine for us," one of them pleaded. "Every time you come in, he gets grumpy and irritable for the whole day. He complains about this foolish patient who never takes any kind of pain medication. He makes our day miserable after you're here."

Even so, I had the procedure without any anesthetic. But the dentist was his usual grumpy, irritable self around me. He continued to insist that I *must* use the Novocaine to avoid "the horrible pain. It must be killing you."

These are not the kind of suggestions you want to hear while using self-hypnosis to avoid the pain a dental drill can inflict. I explained to one of my colleagues at a hypnosis conference—he was a dentist and we were both training through the American Society of Clinical Hypnosis—about my dentist. He smiled.

"Of course he would act that way," he explained. "When he was trained decades ago, he learned that he has to inflict pain to bring about a cure, and also that he's in control of everything happening in his dental operatory."

That made sense to me.

"So find a way to put him in control of your experience of pain," my colleague suggested. "In other words, use hypnosis for his comfort, too."

At my next dental visit, the dentist and I shook hands. Immediately, he warned, "This is really going to hurt. You must take the anesthesia today."

Once again, I declined, but I added, "I have an even stronger way to control pain, but you'll have to do it for me."

He looked puzzled, so I continued.

"Any time you think I need more anesthesia, instead of thinking about how I must use Novocaine, I want you to press my right shoulder."

He reached toward my shoulder, and I said, "Not yet, only when I need to go deeper into trance!"

As he began the procedure, seated on my right, he would periodically press on my shoulder. Sometimes he pressed so hard, it hurt. Then I heard him say to his assistant, "Watch this!" as he pressed on my shoulder and continued drilling. He was delighted that he had the ability to alleviate my pain by pressing my shoulder.

In fact, he became so enthusiastic, he made a suggestion that taught me a powerful lesson.

"Since you're doing so well with the pain," he said, "can you turn off the bleeding?"

In my mind, I imagined a faucet near the tooth undergoing the procedure, and I closed the faucet.

"That's great!" he said. "Now turn off the saliva so I can get this suction device out of my way."

I recalled from only a week earlier a hike in the desert near my home when I hadn't taken enough water and my mouth became very dry. I recalled that feeling, and for good measure, also imagined eating salty potato chips that made my mouth even drier. The dentist pulled the suction device out of my mouth and commended me for also turning off the flow of saliva.

My procedure was completed with not a trace of discomfort, and the dentist was in good spirits and thrilled about controlling my pain.

An important note in this case: The way we experience either our sense of control or our sense of helplessness, along with our beliefs about control and helplessness, make a huge contribution to either our pain or comfort. Although I initially invented the shoulder-squeezing technique to let my dentist feel that he was in control of my comfort, he taught me that I could also control the flow of blood and saliva, which had never entered my mind. Subsequently, I have written articles about clinical hypnosis and surgery, noting that in nearly all the studies, the benefits of hypnosis for surgery include less anxiety beforehand, lesser amounts of anesthesia required during surgery, less fluid loss and better blood flow control during the procedure, less pain medicine needed after surgery, faster or more rapid healing times, lower rates of infection and complications, and shorter hospital stays.

My wife, Joy, has also successfully used hypnosis to control pain during dental procedures. Her dentist told her she would need anesthesia during the procedures required to make a crown, but she said she was going to use hypnosis instead.

I had spent about thirty minutes with her earlier that day, giving her a brief session on going into trance and the many ways she could imagine turning down the nerve sensation in her mouth.

While she was in the chair for forty minutes, she became so relaxed and unconcerned, it felt to her as though the entire procedure had taken only five or ten minutes. The dentist could not understand how she had withstood so much pain. He even called her "super human" for this ability. In reality, she experienced no pain at all. She returned home, proud of herself. "I just went to Mazatlan and sat under the palapa, eating fresh salsa and guacamole, and gazing out over the beautiful Pacific," she told me.

What made hypnosis work so successfully for her? She had a high motivation to be comfortable and to avoid having chemicals injected into her body. She believed it would work because she has witnessed how well hypnosis has worked for my patients over the years. And she knew she would feel much better, both physically and emotionally, having learned to use this mind-body tool to experience dental work while remaining comfortable and in control of her experience.

In almost forty years of practice, I've never had anyone request pain control at the dentist. But I have worked with dozens of people who have come to see me requesting hypnosis to overcome the fear of going to the dentist. And, in every single case, they discovered their ability to relax and produce their own comfort at the dentist's office. A great many learned they did not need to use anesthesia, and the time in the dental chair seemed like minutes. If you don't believe you can do this at your dentist's office, you're not alone. But if you're open to the idea of changing that belief, you'll be amazed by what you can do.

What These Cases Teach Us

All the cases in this chapter demonstrate that pain is a subjective experience. No one can see pain or measure it. We can associate ideas with pain, such as seeing someone drop something heavy on his foot or smash his finger with a hammer. We can read an x-ray and see broken bones. But we cannot see pain. Because it is a subjective experience, we can only perceive it within ourselves.

Pain is also very motivating, for no one wants to experience it. Hypnosis allows us to change or alter our perceptions of pain in a variety of ways. These include substituting one sensation for another, detaching or dissociating from our bodies, altering time, or making friends with the pain. Once you discover your ability to alter your perception by using your imagination, you're also changing your beliefs about what you are experiencing. Remember the vital ingredients that make hypnosis effective—motivation, belief, and expectation—and, most importantly, that your subconscious mind-body cannot tell the difference between what is real and what is imagined.

Chapter 11

Medical Hexing—and Doing the Impossible

Remember that old saying, "Sticks and stones may break my bones, but words can never hurt me"? We now know that words can indeed hurt, sometimes seriously, because of the way the subconscious works. It hears words literally and takes them at face value, even if we do not remember or understand them. The body then reacts accordingly, producing physical symptoms based on the literal meaning of the words. Medical hexing is one way that words can hurt.

I first heard the term *medical hexing* from my friend and colleague Dr. Andrew Weil. It describes the way physicians and other medical professionals can unwittingly hex their patients with language, creating a belief system in the patient that negatively affects the ultimate outcome of the case. (Of course, positive words can also lead to a more positive outcome.)

Often, doctors believe the only ethical course is to tell patients the "truth," such as how long they might expect to live when diagnosed with a serious illness or what side effects they might experience when taking a drug. Yes, it is often a difficult balancing act between being truthful and being optimistic and encouraging. However, in not understanding the power of their words, doctors can cause unnecessary suffering for their patients. In our culture, doctors are the experts we entrust with our health and our lives, so it is difficult for many people to ignore or disagree with them— even if they are not aware of having heard the damaging words.

I've helped many of my patients understand and then undo medical hexing.

A Reason to Panic

One case of medical hexing that stands out in my mind is Sam, who was seventy-one and retired from the auto industry in Detroit when he moved to Tucson. He had begun having panic attacks for what appeared to be no reason, so he made an appointment with me to see if hypnosis would help.

As I took Sam's history, it appeared that he was leading a charmed life here in the desert. Now that he was retired, he had plenty of time to enjoy his new home, and as he said, he particularly enjoyed no longer having to shovel snow off the sidewalk or scrape ice off his windshield. Since he could not identify any stresses, he was confused as to why he would be having panic attacks—moments of sheer terror during which he literally felt as if he were going to die.

I asked Sam about his medical history. About seven or eight years earlier, he had been diagnosed with colorectal cancer and had successfully undergone treatment. He had waited to move to Tucson until he was well past the milestone five-year mark with no recurrence, so he said he was no longer worried about cancer.

We began Sam's treatment with some simple relaxation techniques. Relaxation is the opposite physical response to anxiety, in which the body produces increased heart rate, blood pressure, and muscle tension. In panic attacks like the ones Sam was experiencing, these symptoms are so intense that the sufferer believes death is imminent. The fact that there often appears to be no reason for the attacks only compounds the anxiety, which begins a vicious circle of escalating attacks. Therefore, if Sam could teach his body to relax and produce physical conditions opposite to those associated with panic, he could lessen or eliminate the attacks.

During our first session, Sam had an insight into his anxiety while in trance and practicing relaxation techniques in different parts of his body. In fact, we had not quite finished the instructional part of the session when he stopped, opened his eyes, and said, "I know what it is!"

"Would you like to share it with me?" I asked.

Share he did, with much enthusiasm.

"I moved out here only when I knew I was past the five-year mark for my cancer," he repeated. "But once I was settled, I followed up with an oncologist here. My doctor in Michigan recommended that I do that."

I nodded at the sound advice.

"The oncologist had all these residents with him, so it was like I had an audience for my checkup and tests. The doc says I look perfectly fine, with no traces of cancer, no symptoms whatsoever. He even congratulated me on my wonderful survival. That's what he said—'wonderful survival.' I was happy, but I already knew I was fine."

Sam shook his head as he recalled what happened next. "I got dressed and got on the elevator. Then the doctor and the residents got in. I was jammed way in the back, so when we got to their floor, the last resident to leave before the doors closed looked back at me and said, 'Congratulations. Now all we have to do is wait for the other shoe to drop.'"

I immediately understood the basis for Sam's anxiety.

"And now I remember that my first panic attack was that night," he said, exultant at having solved the puzzle.

We completed our session, and I sent him home with a CD to practice his relaxation skills. He used it for a while to release his fear, but since he now understood the source of the attacks, he never had another one after our session.

The resident's words "hexed" Sam, who previously had been confident about his health after completing his cancer treatment and especially after passing the five-year mark. While he had not consciously recalled those words until our session, nor made the connection to the onset of the panic attacks, they had sown doubt and fear in his subconscious.

Do You Feel Sick Yet?

Medical hexing can also happen to groups of people. It is important for first responders, such as paramedics and police officers, to understand this so they can avoid making a situation worse.

A colleague of mine in Texas, Gary Elkins, PhD, told me about a case of what could be called mass medical hexing at a high school football game. Paramedics were present, as usual, in case of an injury to a football player or spectator. The stands were packed with parents, students, and other residents of the small town.

During the game, one of the cheerleaders became sick to her stomach and had to vomit. Unable to make it to the bathroom, she threw up on the sidelines, which was extremely embarrassing. But after the game was delayed and paramedics rushed to her aid, it became much more than simply embarrassing.

When someone is nauseated and throws up, usually the first question anyone asks is, "What did you eat today?" Which was exactly the question the paramedics posed to the distraught cheerleader, who was one of the most popular girls in the school.

"I had macaroni and cheese at the school cafeteria," she replied.

Since everyone was paying close attention to her situation, her answer spread like wildfire through the stands. One of the paramedics even picked up a megaphone and asked the crowd, "Who ate at the school cafeteria today?" Panic began to spread.

Soon after the ambulance delivered the cheerleader to the emergency room, at least twenty-five other students arrived there, saying they, too, were feeling nauseated because they had also eaten the cafeteria's mac and cheese. As it turned out, none of them were very sick at all, and there was no mass case of food poisoning.

However, there had been a case of mass medical hexing, which began with the paramedic asking the crowd about their lunch choices that day. Our minds are naturally suggestible, and even the suggestion of symptoms can be contagious.

In my years of practice, I have learned to ask patients about the words they recall hearing during medical situations: when they go to the emergency room, when first responders tend to them at an accident scene, or even when doctors and nurses speak to them during exams, testing, and treatment. Often, they don't recall the frightening messages they received until they are in trance, as Sam did. But once they have made the connection, often all they need is to reframe and restate the words in a more positive way to begin the healing.

Picture This

Even when a condition is caused by an outside force and considered irreversible by conventional medicine, there is hope as long as the person has motivation, belief, and expectation.

A car accident had left Tom, forty-two, with back pain, so he came to see me for help in relieving it. His physician had already determined that no underlying problem would be masked by his use of hypnosis. I could see that Tom was curious and eager to learn, so we talked in some depth about how I had seen hypnosis help many of my patients relieve pain from many sources.

When I took Tom's medical history, as I do with all my patients, he mentioned that before the accident he had undergone radiation therapy for bone cancer on his hip. He showed me the area where the focused and repeated radiation had severely damaged the skin, leaving a large patch of leathery scar tissue. This increased his back pain because the hard, inflexible skin prevented him from bending or twisting at the hip.

"My radiation oncologist's last words to me were that I have to learn to live with it," Tom explained. "He said there's no way to renew or replace that damaged skin. It's impossible."

In three sessions, I taught Tom self-hypnosis so he could relax his back muscles and, in the process, reduce the pain. He did very well, and his success increased his interest in hypnosis and healing, so I lent him an excellent book on the subject.

About two years later, I pulled the same book off the shelf to hand to Arlene, a gynecologist with her office in the same medical complex as mine. She had come over to ask me a few questions about hypnosis, interested in how it might help some of her patients.

She began flipping through the book and then gasped, a look of embarrassed surprise covering her face.

"Is this you?" she asked warily.

I had no idea what she was talking about.

She held up two Polaroid photographs that had been sandwiched inside the book—photos of a naked man in profile from knee to armpit, with genitals clearly visible.

I was stunned as well as embarrassed.

"I don't understand this," I managed to say.

Arlene studied the photos. "Look. In one of the pictures, there's a dark brown patch on his hip, and in the other one, there isn't."

I immediately realized who the man in the photos was.

When I saw Tom a little while later and told him about my experience with Arlene, he laughed.

"I was wondering when you would find those," he said, still grinning. "I didn't mean to embarrass you."

"Well, once I saw the dark patch on the one and not on the other, I figured out who it was."

"If you think you were shocked, you should have seen my radiation oncologist," said Tom. "He was floored. He couldn't believe I'd been able to grow new skin over that spot. He was pretty impressed."

Tom explained that his success with his back pain gave him the idea to try self-hypnosis on the patch of skin.

"Every morning after my shower, I'd stand in front of the mirror and look at both hips and pictured healthy skin on the right one, just like I had on the left one. The healing sort of happened automatically. By the end of the year, I had grown new skin."

He had taken the "before" and "after" photos as a form of proof.

"I'm sorry you were embarrassed," he repeated, still chuckling. "But it's amazing, isn't it?"

Tom was not the only beneficiary of his hypnosis training. Arlene was so impressed with Tom's healing that she took professional training in medical hypnosis so she could offer it to her patients.

What These Cases Teach Us

The message I would like you take away from this chapter is that words can hurt or words can heal, but they are only words, so they can be changed. It is important for you to step back and look at the words in question with conscious awareness. Then you can decide whether those words were spoken to you in error by a medical professional or if they are appropriate for you. Remember that *Hypnosis House Call* is about how to use words, ideas, intentions, and beliefs in a way that is beneficial for you. With this knowledge, you can use self-hypnosis to gain control of your health.

When Richard H. Carmona, MD, former U.S. surgeon general, was chief of trauma and air rescue here in Tucson, he asked me to make a presentation at an in-service training for his team of first responders about the words they should use on scene. Later, some colleagues and I created a video with similar information for first responders. We taught them that their first words to a victim at a trauma scene should be, "Help is on the way [or here now] and I'm going to stay with you. You can let yourself relax now. Everything is going to be fine." Saying these words in a calm, reassuring manner can neutralize fear and help minimize trauma and pain.

PART III

Healing Your Mind–Body with Hypnosis

This final part of *Hypnosis House Call* focuses on healing your mind-body through hypnosis. If we were together during a session, I could "tailor" your hypnosis experience for you. I would ask you questions and gather information pertinent to you. Instead, you will provide the information through a series of questions. And you will be your own therapist. The questions will stimulate thoughts about things personal to you. You will be directed to use this information to analyze your reason for using hypnosis, to formulate positive hypnotic suggestions, and to incorporate these suggestions into trance. Finally, you will be able to practice your self-hypnosis by yourself or with the trancework on the DVD.

Chapter 12

Tailoring Your Hypnosis

By now you have become acquainted with me and my work in using hypnosis to alleviate a variety of common conditions. You have learned about the mind-body connection and how hypnosis can let you use the power of your mind for healing and other benefits.

Now it is time for your specific application. Here are some questions I want you to answer for me:

- Where were you born and raised?

- Where did you go to school and what did you study?

- What kinds of jobs have you had?

- What hobbies and interests have given you pleasure through your life?

- What places and times did you feel the best about yourself and about what you were doing?

- Did you learn to play a musical instrument?

- What are your hobbies and interests now?

- If you had all the time and money to study or pursue an interest, what would you do?

- What kind of pets did you have, or do you have now?

– What colors do you like?

– What season of the year gives you a good feeling?

– Can you remember places and times when you
experienced daydreaming, like school or meetings?

– Do you already have a favorite place you go to in
imagination to feel safe and good?

In this Hypnosis House Call, we will begin by hearing "your story." You can write it or speak it as if I were with you right now. Follow these steps.

1. Imagine that I am present with you right now.
You would hear me ask, "Tell me your story." I
would ask you all these questions, which you can
answer now for yourself.

– What symptoms are you experiencing?

– When did the symptoms begin?

– Did they come on suddenly or gradually?

– What examinations and diagnoses have you
obtained from your doctor or specialist?

– How do these medical professionals explain it
to you?

– Describe the symptoms and conditions as you
experience them, as richly and fully as possible.
I often ask my patients to "describe what you
experience so well that I would be able to feel what
you feel, as if I had it myself."

– What was going on in your life during the six
months before symptoms first began to appear?

– What is your intuitive belief about how this condition happened or evolved?

2. Analyze what you are experiencing. I know it is difficult to separate yourself from what you are going through, but do your best to be an objective observer of all you have described in #1 above.

– What metaphors or words give meaning to what you feel with these symptoms or conditions?

– Give some thought to the metaphors someone outside your body would use to describe or summarize what is going on with you. For example: He's beside himself; she's just burning up over that; he's really a pain in the neck, etc.

3. Now, let's formulate some positive statements that express what you *want* (not what you *don't want*). Specifically, what would you like to have instead of the symptoms? Here are several examples. For skin: My skin is smooth and clear. For GI: My stomach is calm and relaxed. For headache: My scalp is relaxed, my forehead is smooth, my neck and shoulders relax and I let my pillow hold all the weight of my head, and my hands are warm. For stress: My nerves are calm, my mind is relaxed, I am safe, all is well, and I am at peace.

Say these statements aloud, but know that it is also helpful to write them down. One of my teachers, Milton Erickson, advised writing down and revising the hypnotic suggestion enough times so that you distill the suggestion down to its most clear, succinct, and positive message. (When I do this exercise, I have found myself writing out pages, line after line, until reaching the most positive, accurate message of what I want my mind-body to accept.)

In addition to words, use your imagination to create the image of what you want, just as if it has already happened. Picture it as clearly and perfectly as you like. Do not worry about "how" to make it happen. Just focus on the image of it happening or already being accomplished.

4. Now, select one of the hypnotic induction methods specified in Chapter 3. Use it to shift your attention within you—shift your attention into imagination. Become absorbed with your thoughts and images. Remember the questions I asked you about yourself, such as where you grew up, what pets you have, and so on? Use your answers to these questions to embellish what you are imagining. Draw on your personal images and pleasant memories, and incorporate them into this imaginative experience. In other words, use the answers from your personal life to embellish and enrich the images in order to tailor this trance more personally for you.

You will be aware of where you are and what is going on around you. But you will also notice that your attention is more focused within you. And now you can deepen your focus within.

Now, recall the suggestions you wrote down. Repeat the suggestions as a statement of TRUTH within yourself. Pretend or imagine that your subconscious mind is accepting these ideas, accepting the intention of your message. Let your subconscious use everything you have learned and experienced to make it happen for you.

If you like, imagine that your subconscious is like a waiter or waitress taking your order to the chef. Be sure that your language and instructions are exactly what you do want.

Or imagine that you are the captain of a large ship standing on the bridge so you are able to see in all directions and can choose where you want to go. You are giving messages to the powerhouse in the engine room beneath the waterline; it has no windows and simply follows your commands explicitly.

The message has been delivered. Let it go . . . allow your subconscious to act on it for you. Your work is done after stating what you want.

Now turn ON your imagination and create the scene or picture of having what you want . . . see it as it is done, completed perfectly to your satisfaction. Imagine yourself enjoying what you have received. Imagine how good you feel now that you have received exactly what you asked for. Picture it, experience it, feel it. Give thanks or simply feel the gratification within you.

When you are ready, remind yourself that it is done and your subconscious (the mind of your body) has received and accepted the idea as you intended it. Rest assured that it is happening now as you shift over to bring yourself to an alert waking state, feeling comfortably in a fully waking state.

5. Practice your hypnosis once or twice a day. Also use the DVD to let me help you accomplish this. You'll discover how rapidly the experience becomes familiar to you and how it becomes easier and easier to achieve, and easier to repeat with greater ease and confidence. Spend as little or as much time as you like doing your self-hypnosis, and make it pleasant to do.

Sooner or later you will discover the changes that are happening. The order of the changes does not matter. Your mind-body delivers what you desire in the very best way for you.

A Final Word

This completes your Hypnosis House Call. Use the DVD enclosed with this book to reinforce your practice as needed. You will discover that with regular use *your* talents for using *your* hypnosis continue to improve. As I mentioned throughout this house call, all hypnosis is self-hypnosis. If you have allowed yourself to do the exercises in the book and on the DVD, you are now well prepared to use your hypnosis to enjoy the benefits of mind-body healing.

With the understanding you have gained through this house call, you are also ready to proceed in reviewing and using other hypnosis-related materials that are available for specific purposes. Think of yourself as being way ahead of the game when it comes to using hypnosis for your needs and desires.

Acknowledgments

Hypnosis House Call did not happen by itself. I want to first acknowledge and thank the patients who came to see me and trusted me to help them use hypnosis for healing. In almost forty years of practice, it is you, the patients, who have given me the greatest rewards for my efforts and sustained my love affair with hypnotic healing.

I also want to thank Barbara Stahura for sharing her writing wisdom, literary coaching, and friendship to help me write. Jim Pavett is a professional drummer, audio engineer, and gifted producer, who stepped up to the plate to make the DVD happen. And thanks also to Terry McKee for such timely turnaround in transcription and typing.

Likewise, I am grateful to my editors, Kate Zimmermann and Michael Fragnito at Sterling Publishing, for giving me the opportunity to put this book in your hands in such fine form.

My literary agent, Arthur Klebanoff, deserves a medal for his fortitude and loyalty in bringing *hypnosis* out, despite many voices arguing to change the word to make it acceptable to the marketplace. When shopping for an agent, Mr. Klebanoff impressed my wife and me the moment we met him. His intellectual brilliance and creativity keep me in awe. Thank you, Arthur.

I am indebted to my first wife, Jody, for many rich years of loving bliss. Our time together was much too short. And I thank her for giving me our daughter, Elise, whom I cherish and admire. I still hear Elise's young voice when I gripe about an ache or pain, reminding me, "Why don't you use your hypnosis, Dad?"

Dr. Andrew Weil is both a friend and a hero of mine. His dedication to improving medical education and bringing natural healing with integrative medicine to the public has been a beacon of light to my own journey "against the grain" of the medical mainstream. Thank goodness for Dr. Weil, for uplifting the face of medicine and for his thoughtful words in the foreword to this book.

My wife, Joy, is truly the joy in my life and my partner in all things wonderful. You have helped me in more ways than I can count, and more than you realize. Your loving support is such a blessing to me. I cannot fully express how much your intelligence, beauty, compassion, and amazing practical skills make *me* happen.

History of Hypnosis

The term *hypnosis* has been around since the 1840s, but healers began using this technique, or some form of it, centuries earlier. We have records of hypnosis going back 2,500 years in ancient China and Egypt. In ancient Greece, the physical remnants of the sleep-healing temple of Asklepios still exist.

Asklepios, the Greek god of physicians, created a sleep-healing temple where people would enter a dimly lit stone room (called an Abaton) and recline on a stone bench that was elevated on one end, much like a chaise longue. (This bench was called a klini, which is the origin of our word *clinic*.) The patients were prepared for several days in advance with purifying waters, baths, and fasting. They learned to relax into a peaceful calm. Then, on the day of their treatment, they would enter the Abaton. They were instructed to recline on the klini, to enter their calm reverie, and to silently await Asklepios. He would then come into the chamber and whisper his intention to them, based on their illness or condition. He might say, "I'm going to take your headaches away" or "You can eat anything you want now, free of discomfort" or "You will sleep well now." After his gentle touch and affirmative words, he would then leave. We believe his treatments worked because his patients carved testimonials into the stones and rocks around the temple, telling of their cures.

Although not yet known as *hypnosis,* this kind of treatment continued throughout history, from practitioners such as the Persian physician Avicenna around AD 1000, the Swiss physician Paracelsus in the sixteenth century, and others. Yet the person who had the most influence on modern hypnotism was Franz Anton Mesmer, an Austrian physician who lived from 1734 to 1815. Around 1770, he began investigating what was then called "animal magnetism"—the practice of using magnets to move energy around people to heal them. (It had nothing to do with animals; instead, *animal* referred to sentient beings, as opposed to the vegetable and mineral classes.) In one reported experiment, Mesmer cut a patient and after he passed a magnet over the wound, the bleeding stopped. However, the bleeding also stopped when he used a stick of wood instead of a magnet. In time, he created trance-inducing methods, including touching and stroking patients, as well as staring into their eyes and waving magnetic wands that he believed would remedy the "cosmic fluid imbalance" in their bodies. He was convinced that these techniques could banish illness and suffering, and they often did if the patient was susceptible to this "mesmerism."

Mesmer became very popular, and he let this go to his head. He grew eccentric, wearing capes and gowns decorated with stars and crescent moons, and often made a spectacle of himself by waving around an iron rod. In 1784, other physicians petitioned King Louis XVI of France to investigate Mesmer and his techniques, to which many people of the time objected. Louis appointed a commission to do this work; it included Benjamin Franklin, who then lived in France; the chemist Antoine Lavoisier; and Dr. Joseph-Ignace Guillotin, the peaceable man for whom the guillotine was later, and unfortunately, named. The commission ultimately ruled that Mesmer's methods had no medical value—remember that medical practices at the time included "scientific" methods such as bloodletting and applying leeches—and Mesmer was discredited.

However, other French and British physicians in the mid-1800s who were interested in the results Mesmer obtained with his patients studied his work and techniques. They eventually discovered that whatever healing occurred was not the result of anything magnetic but because of the power of suggestion. Mesmer's patients, whom he was able to induce into a very relaxed, dreamlike state, responded to his suggestions; their bodies responded in some unknown way that healed their condition or illness. This discovery led the British doctor John Elliotson, who was president of the Royal Medical and Chirurgical [Surgical] Society of London to become more interested in mesmerism. He founded and edited a magazine called *The Zoist* about this new technique, but he, too, was ridiculed because of his interest in it. However, Elliotson also introduced the stethoscope to England, and that became a long-lasting tool of medicine.

Many believe that in 1843, James Braid, a Scottish surgeon, coined the term *hypnosis* based on Hypnos, the Greek god of sleep, in the mistaken notion that someone in a hypnotic trance is asleep. However, my distinguished colleague, Dr. Melvin Gravitz, a noted authority on the history of hypnosis, tells me that the term *hypnosis* was first used by the French physician Etienne Félix d'Henin de Cuvillers. While many physicians continued to discount hypnosis, a number of others began investigating it. Sigmund Freud studied it around 1885, and used it for a time, but then abandoned it in favor of conscious psychoanalysis.

In 1920, Emile Coué, a French pharmacist, wrote the first book on "autosuggestion," or self-hypnosis, titled *Self Mastery through Conscious Autosuggestion*. He had long given his patients affirmations, or positive statements, to say as a daily ritual, in the belief that these suggestions would improve their lives and health. His most famous affirmation is, "Every day in every way, I am getting better and better." In his book, he offered other instructions about self-hypnosis, including the warning, "Never the nots." This is a warning to use only positive statements in self-hypnosis because the subconscious mind cannot recognize a negative statement. For instance, if you say, "I do not want to smoke," your subconscious hears, "I want to smoke," and you act accordingly, puzzled as to why your interest in cigarettes is not diminishing.

The modern study of hypnosis began with psychologist Clark Hull. In his book, *Hypnosis and Suggestibility,* published in 1933, he offered a rigorous examination of hypnosis. He determined that hypnosis was not sleep and had no connection with it. His work also reined in hypnotists' extravagant claims and demonstrated the reality of pain reduction through hypnotic trance. He clearly showed that effects of hypnosis were the result of suggestion and motivation. Hull is famous for the way he stared into the eyes of his patients until they became hypnotically induced.

Thanks to Hull's work, many wounded soldiers in World War II were treated for pain successfully with hypnosis when morphine was not available. These results led to the creation of the Society for Clinical and Experimental Hypnosis in 1949, now an international organization of "psychologists, psychiatrists, social workers, nurses, dentists, and physicians who are dedicated to the highest level of scientific inquiry and the conscientious application of hypnosis in the clinical setting." In 1957, Dr. Milton Erickson and others created the American Society for Clinical Hypnosis. Both of these professional societies share and have similar memberships, yet the former focuses more on experimental research and the latter on clinical applications of hypnosis. The American Society of Clinical Hypnosis is now the organization that provides the certification in clinical hypnosis. This certification is much more professional than the certifications from other schools awarded to people who do not have degrees in medicine, psychology, dentistry, social work, psychotherapy, or nursing.

Better research methods and technologies in recent years have brought mind-body medicine and hypnosis more into the public eye. With neuroimaging devices, such as functional MRIs and PET scans, we can see inside the brain to view in real time what is happening when someone is pretending, imagining, or responding to hypnotic suggestion. What we have found is that the brain cannot tell the difference between what is real and what is only imagined. The brain responds as if the event were actually happening: When a person imagines a cat, the brain acts as if a cat were actually present. If a person is given a hypnotic suggestion that something painful is happening to her foot, the portion of the brain that senses pain in the foot "lights up," just as if the pain were real.

An interesting study about color was done with people in a hypnotic trance. While they were in this state, it was suggested to them that they were looking at a black-white-gray scale when, in fact, they had a full-color scale in front of their eyes. However, the part of the brain that manages monochrome images became very active, while the part of the brain that manages color remained quiet. These results, and others, give much credibility to the powers of hypnosis and suggestion.

I believe we're on the verge of many more and greater discoveries in the field of neuroplasticity, or the brain's ability to reorganize itself according to various stimuli. As studies performed with Tibetan monks and other long-time meditators have shown, brain changes occur in response to meditation done over long periods. Many other studies have demonstrated that exercises, activities, and even thoughts cause physical changes in the brain. We are indeed what we think!

In large part, the same thing happens with hypnosis—we change based on what we tell our brains, or, more accurately, what we tell the subconscious mind so that the physical brain reacts accordingly. With hypnosis and other methods, we use the power of our minds to physically influence our brains for healing and enhancement of body, mind, and spirit.

Resources

Finding a Qualified Practitioner

The American Society of Clinical Hypnosis (ASCH) bestows two levels of certification on professional practitioners of clinical hypnosis: *Certified* and *Approved Consultant. Certified* is bestowed after a required number of hours of study in specified areas and after two years of clinical experience, including supervision. *Approved Consultant* is bestowed after additional hours of study and after five years of clinical practice.

ASCH offers a referral service of qualified practitioners at its Web site, www.asch.net.

The Society for Clinical and Experimental Hypnosis (www.sceh. us) is another distinguished professional association, which also provides training in clinical hypnosis.

SCEH and ASCH share approximately 80 percent of the same members. However, SCEH is more focused on experimental research studies of hypnosis, whereas ASCH is more oriented to clinical applications as well.

Books about Hypnosis

Bristol, Claude M. *The Magic of Believing.* New York: Pocket Books, 1948/1991.

Coué, Emile. *Self Mastery through Conscious Autosuggestion.* WhiteFish, Mont.: Kessinger Publishing, 1997.

Crasilneck. Harold B., and James A. Hall. *Clinical Hypnosis: Principles and Applications,* 2nd ed. Orlando, Fla: Grune and Stratton, 1985.

Hammond, D. Corydon. *Handbook of Hypnotic Suggestions and Metaphors.* New York: W. W. Norton & Co., 1990.

Kroger, William. *Clinical and Experimental Hypnosis*. Philadelphia: J. B. Lippincott Co, 1963.

Lee, Roberta. *The SuperStress Solution*. New York: Random House, 2010.

Lipton, Bruce H. *The Biology of Belief: Unleashing the Power of Consciousness, Matter, and Miracles*. Santa Rosa, Calif: Mountain of Love, 2005.

Low Dog, Tieraona, and Maizes, V. (Eds.). *Integrative Women's Health*. Oxford University Press, 2010.

Meyer, Robert G. *Practical Clinical Hypnosis: Techniques and Practice*. New York: Lexington Books, 1992.

Olness, Karen, and Daniel P. Kohen. *Hypnosis and Hypnotherapy with Children*. 3rd ed. New York: Guilford Press, 1996.

Pelletier, Kenneth R. *Sound Mind, Sound Body: A New Model for Lifelong Health*. New York: Fireside, 1995.

Rakel, David (Ed.). *Integrative Medicine (3rd Edition)*. Saunders, Elsevier, 2011.

Rosen, Sidney, ed. *My Voice Will Go with You: The Teaching Tales of Milton Erickson*. New York: W. W. Norton & Co., 1982.

Rosenfeld, Marc. *A Critical History of Hypnotism, the UNauthorized Story*. Xlibiris Corporation, 2008.

Rossi, Ernest L., and David B. Cheek. *Mind-Body Therapy: Methods of Ideodynamic Healing in Hypnosis*. New York: W. W. Norton & Co., 1988.

Rossman, Martin. *The Worry Solution*. New York: Random House, 2010.

Schneider, Jennifer. *Living with Chronic Pain, 2nd ed*. Healthy Living Books, Hatherleigh Press, 2009.

Schubiner, Howard. *Unlearn Your Pain.* Mind Body Publishing, 2010.

Spiegel, Herbert, and David Spiegel. *Trance and Treatment: Clinical Uses of Hypnosis,* 2nd ed. Washington, D.C.: American Psychiatric Publishing, 2004.

Temes, Roberta. *The Complete Idiot's Guide to Hypnosis,* 2nd ed. New York: Alpha Books, 2004.

Zeig, Jeffrey K., ed. *Ericksonian Approaches to Hypnosis and Psychotherapy.* New York: Brunner/Mazel, 1982.

Other Titles by Dr. Steven Gurgevich

Website: http://www.HealingWithHypnosis.com
Over 60 titles in the "Healing with Hypnosis" and "Hypnotic Tonics" series of hynosis applications.

Heal Yourself with Medical Hypnosis (coauthor, Andrew Weil, MD). 2-CD set. Boulder, Colo.: Sounds True, Inc., 2005.

The Self-Hypnosis Home Study Course. 16-CD set/107-page workbook. Boulder, Colo.: Sounds True, Inc., 2005.

The Self-Hypnosis Diet. 3-CD set. Boulder, Colo.: Sounds True, Inc., 2006.

The Self-Hypnosis Diet. 214-page book & CD. Boulder, Colo.: Sounds True, Inc., 2007/2009.

Relieve Anxiety with Medical Hypnosis. 2-CD set. Boulder, Colo.: Sounds True, Inc., 2007.

Relax Rx. 2-CD set. Boulder, Colo.: Sounds True, Inc., 2008.

Deep Sleep with Medical Hypnosis. 2-CD set. Boulder, Colo.: Sounds True, Inc., 2009.

Relieve Stress with Medical Hypnosis. 2-CD set. Boulder, Colo.: Sounds True, Inc., 2010.

Index

A

Abaton, 177

A Critical History of Hypnotism, the Unauthorized Story, 184

Age progression, 22

Age repression, 22

Alerting, 42

American Society of Clinical Hypnosis

author's involvement with, 6, 7

definition of hypnosis, 9

and history of hypnosis, 180

Amnesia, as effect of hypnosis, 22

"Animal magnetism," 177, 178

Approved Consultant, 183

Arizona Center for Integrative Medicine, 6, 49

Arm levitation, 36, 37, 38

Asklepios, 177

Avicenna, 177

B

Back pain

and medical hexing, 161, 162, 163

treating with angels and saints, 141, 142

Bannister, Roger, 26

Belief, importance of, 19, 20

"Belly brain," 83

The Biology of Belief: Unleashing the Power of Consciousness, 184

Bone cancer, and chemotherapy, treating with hypnosis, 126, 127, 128

Braid, James, 179

Brain plasticity, 14

Breathing and breath induction, 38, 39

Bristo, Claude, 183

"Broken heart syndrome," 19, 99

Buckets and balloons, 31

C

Cardiovascular system, treating with hypnosis

cases, lessons from, 105

heartbreak, 101, 102–103

hypertension and congestive heart failure, 99, 100–101

white-coat hypertension, 103, 104, 105

Catalepsy, as effect of hypnosis, 22

Certified Consultant, 183

Children and hypnosis, 25, 53

Clinical and Experimental Hypnosis, 183

Clinical hypnosis. *See also* Hypnosis

professional practitioners of, 183

versus "everyday" hypnosis, 10

versus stage hypnosis, 13

Clinical Hypnosis: Principles and Applications, 183

Colitis, treating with hypnosis, 83, 84–88, 89

Color, study on, 180, 181

Coming out of trance, 42

The Complete Idiot's Guide to Hypnosis, 185

Congestive heart failure, treating with hypnosis, 99, 100–101

Conscious mind

description of, 13

and differences with the unconscious mind, 5

COPD, treating with hypnosis, 79, 80–81

Corneal transplants, 132–134, 135

Neuroplasticity, 14, 181

The New England Journal of Medicine, 21

No-induction induction, 41

Not, use of word in hypnosis, 17

"Notes of a Biology Watcher," 21

O

Olness, Karen, 184

P

Pain, controlling with hypnosis
  cases, lessons from 155, 156
  dentistry, 151, 152–154, 155
  headaches, from accident, 147, 148–150
  headaches, common, 150, 151
  fractured pubic bone and pelvis, 142, 143
  inguinal groin hernia, 143, 144
  migraines, 137, 138–140, 141
  multiple fractures, 144, 145–146
  ruptured discs in back, 141, 142

Pancreatitis, treating with hypnosis, 95, 96

Panic attacks
  author's experience with, 5
  and medical hexing, 158, 159, 160

Paracelsus, 177

Patient cases of treatment with hypnosis
  asthma, 74–78, 79
  back pain, 141, 142, 161, 162, 163
  blindness, 132, 133–134, 135
  bone cancer, loss of appetite from, 126, 127–128
  car accident victim, 144, 145–146
  COPD, 79, 80, 81
  dentistry, 151, 152–153, 154

  difficulty swallowing, 91, 92, 93
  erectile dysfunction, 115, 116–117
  fertility, 108, 109–110
  fibroids, 110, 111, 112
  fractured public bone and pelvis, 142, 143
  headache, common, 150, 151
  headache, from operation, 147–149, 150
  heartbreak, 101, 102, 103
  hyperemesis gravidarum, 112, 113–114, 115
  hypertension and congestive heart failure, 99, 100, 100, 101
  ileostomy, 93, 94, 95
  inguinal groin hernia, 143, 144
  lymphatic system, 124, 125, 126
  mass medical hexing, 160, 161
  migraine pain, 137, 138–140, 141
  multiple myeloma cancer, 128, 129–131
  nausea and vomiting, 89, 90, 91
  panic attacks, 158–159, 160
  psychoneuroimmunology, 119
  recurrent pancreatic, 95, 96
  scleroderma, 120–123, 124
  shingles, 67, 68–71
  threads in, 49, 50
  ulcerative colitis, 83, 84–88, 89
  warts, 52–66, 67
  white-coat hypertension, 103, 104, 105

Pelletier, Kenneth, 184

Pencil grip, 30, 31

Polio, injections for, 5

Positron emission tomography, VIII

Positive hallucination, as effect of hypnosis, 24

Posthypnotic suggestions
  as effect of hypnosis, 24, 25
  use of in hypnosis, 46

Post-traumatic stress disorder, 91

T

U

V

W

Z

About the Author

Dr. Steven Gurgevich is a licensed psychologist specializing in Mind-Body Medicine. He is a clinical faculty member at the University of Arizona, College of Medicine within Dr. Andrew Weil's Arizona Center for Integrative Medicine. He has been the Director of the Mind-Body Clinic within the integrative medicine center since 1997. He is an approved consultant, fellow, and faculty member of the American Society of Clinical Hypnosis, where he has trained thousands of professionals. He has presented and published numerous professional papers and textbook chapters about the mind-body connection and medical hypnosis.

Dr. Gurgevich founded Tranceformation Works in 1996 to provide hypnosis audios for a variety of medical applications, and is now the author of over 60 titles through his "Healing with Hypnosis" series and "Hypnotic Tonics" available from his website at www.HealingwithHypnosis.com.

Dr. Gurgevich's work has also been published by Sounds True, Inc. This work includes: The Self-Hypnosis Home Study Course; Relax Rx; Relieve Anxiety with Medical Hypnosis; Deep Sleep; Relieve Stress with Medical Hypnosis; The Self-Hypnosis Diet (audio); *The Self-Hypnosis Diet* (book, co-author Joy Gurgevich); and *Heal Yourself with Medical Hypnosis* (co-author Andrew Weil, MD).

Dr. Gurgevich continues his thirty-eight years of private practice at Behavioral Medicine, Ltd. and Sabino Canyon Integrative Medicine, LLC, in Tucson, Arizona. And, *yes*, he is still making house calls.